FUNDAMENTALS OF ONCOLOGY

Henry C. Pitot

McArdle Laboratory for Cancer Research
University of Wisconsin Medical School
Madison, Wisconsin

MARCEL DEKKER, INC.   New York and Basel

Library of Congress Cataloging in Publication Data

Pitot, Henry C.   [Date]
    Fundamentals of oncology

    Includes index.
    1. Cancer. 2. Oncology. I. Title. [DNLM:
1. Neoplasms. QZ200 P685f]
RC261.P57   616.9'92   77-15779
ISBN 0-8247-6677-6

Marcel Dekker, Inc.
270 Madison Avenue, New York, New York 10016

Current printing (last digit):
10 9 8 7 6 5 4 3 2 1

PRINTED IN THE UNITED STATES OF AMERICA

To Mary and Julie

Preface

The sensationalism and publicity directed toward the investigation, diagnosis, and treatment of cancer as a disease in the human being have reached a dramatic level in the United States. In part this is a result of the decision by the political administration of Richard M. Nixon to make the conquest of cancer a major goal of his office. Although it is not my desire nor is this the place to consider the ramifications of this decision and the subsequent difficulties that have arisen in its implementation, it is clear that cancer research received a "shot in the arm" of international proportions by political decisions at the beginning of this decade. The U.S. public, who have supported the National Cancer Plan through their taxes, have been repeatedly apprised of its existence and progress since its inception in 1970. Much has been written on the subject of cancer in the scientific literature as a direct result of the financial impetus given to research in oncology over the past decade. A variety of books and monographs on the general subject of cancer in humans and animals for both the scientist and the layman have appeared during this same period.

This text is not meant to be a popular account of the cancer problem. More than two decades ago, the Department of Oncology, which comprises the McArdle Laboratory for Cancer Research of the University of Wisconsin at Madison, initiated a graduate course in oncology. This course consisted of a series of lectures covering a variety of aspects of experimental oncology including chemical and biological carcinogenesis, host-tumor relationships, the natural history of cancer, and the biochemistry of cancer. In addition, within a few years of its inception, several lectures were given on the diagnosis and therapy of cancer in the human patient. The course was and always has been oriented primarily toward the graduate student in oncology rather than specifically for the medical student or postgraduate physician. In part as a result of the increased interest in cancer research by both graduate and undergraduate students and as part of the mechanism of self-evaluation of teaching programs, several years ago the McArdle Laboratory expanded its original course into three separate courses in experimental oncology. The first course in this series is open to all students and fellows at the University of Wisconsin, and the notes given to the students comprise the basis for this short text on the "fundamentals of oncology."

During the course period, these notes are supplemented by several sessions in which slides are shown depicting a variety of examples both from human and animal neoplasms to illustrate many of the specific points presented in the text. A list of these slides can be made available to anyone interested, on written request to the author. In addition, at the end of the course several lectures are given to the students on the diagnosis and therapy of human cancer as well as on the psychosocial aspects and bioethics of human oncology.

It is the hope of those of us in the McArdle Laboratory involved in the teaching of this course that we can instill in our students the basic concepts of the science of this disease and thereby interest them in learning more about the mechanisms of neoplastic disease and the use of such knowledge toward the ultimate control of cancer in the human patient.

In particular, I would like to express my appreciation to my colleagues in the McArdle Laboratory, especially Drs. James and Elizabeth Miller, Van R. Potter, Ilse Riegel, Bill Sugden, Howard Temin, and others who have read and made critical comments on this manuscript at its earlier stages. My thanks also go to the several outside reviewers of the manuscript whose suggestions resulted in an increased number of illustrations and the addition of the epilog, and to Mr. John L. Shane, whose artistic skill produced the drawings of the figures.

McArdle Laboratory for Cancer Research
University of Wisconsin Medical School
Madison, Wisconsin

Contents

1

Cancer: Yesterday and Today

Throughout history at various periods certain diseases have been most feared by humans. In ancient biblical times the disease which was most feared and abhorred by the general population was leprosy. During the medieval and Renaissance periods in Europe, the dreaded disease was bubonic plague or the "black death." During the nineteenth century the major killer which was associated with the most human suffering was the "white death" or tuberculosis. In the twentieth century and especially as a result of the advances of the sciences, microbiology and pharmacology, infectious diseases do not play the major role in the "developed cultures" that they did in the past. Today the disease that strikes fear in the hearts of most laymen is cancer. One of the more succinct descriptions emphasizing the impact of the fear of the disease was written by Glenn Frank, President of the University of Wisconsin, in 1936 at a symposium on cancer given at the University of Wisconsin School of Medicine.

> But not all these tragic consequences together are the worst evil wrought by cancer. For *everybody* that is *killed* by the *fact* of cancer, multiplied thousands of *minds* are *unnerved* by the *fear* of cancer. What cancer, as an unsolved mystery, does to the morale of millions who may never know its ravages is incalculable. This is an incidence of cancer that cannot be reached by the physician's medicaments, the surgeon's knife, or any organized advice against

panic. Nothing but the actual conquest of cancer itself will re-
move this sword that today hangs over every head.*

Cancer as a disease presents interesting paradoxes. While the layman
looks upon it as perhaps the ultimate horror of all diseases ending in painful,
suffering death, the physician views cancer as another general type of disease
such as inflammation, trauma, toxic or degenerative disease. Many consider
cancer as a multitude of different diseases with an underlying biological kin-
ship. To the experimentalist working in cancer research, the cancer cell results
from one or more derangements in the biological chemistry of a normal cell.

In 1970 a special panel of consultants called together by the U.S.
Senate submitted a report on "A National Program for the Conquest of
Cancer." Although the United States was not the first country to make the
conquest of cancer a national effort, the financial backing requested and
ultimately passed by the executive and legislative branches of government,
respectively, gave the greatest single impetus in the history of this country to
the scientific search for knowledge and understanding of the control and
elimination of cancer. This committee of consultants generated a report
which at that time was perhaps the best summary of the status of cancer as a
disease and of cancer research in this country. This report showed that cancer
is in fact the primary health concern of the people of the United States. In a
number of polls, approximately two-thirds of those questioned admitted fear-
ing cancer more than any other diesease. Of 200 million Americans living in
1970, 50 million were destined to develop cancer at the then present rate of
incidence, and some 34 million would die of the disease. About one-half of all
deaths due to cancer occur prior to the age of 65, and cancer causes more
deaths among children under the age of 15 than any other disease. Since more
than 16% of all deaths in this country are caused by cancer, it is second only
to cardiovascular disease as the greatest killer of our population.

The committee pointed out that in 1969 the budget of this country,
calculated on a per capita basis, enlisted $410 for national defense; $125 for
the war in Viet Nam; $19 for the space program; $19 for foreign aid; but only
89 cents for cancer research. During the same year, deaths from cancer were
eight times the number of lives lost in all six years of the Viet Nam war up to
that time, 5-1/2 times the number of people killed in automobile accidents in

*Quoted from the welcome by President Glenn Frank to participants in "A
Symposium on Cancer," University of Wisconsin School of Medicine, Madison, Wisconsin, Sept. 7-9, 1936. University of Wisconsin Press, Madison: 1938.

that year, and greater than the number of American servicemen killed in battle in all four years of World War II. Literally billions of dollars are lost each year to this nation's economy as a direct result of the ravages of this disease.

This report also emphasized certain other points in relation to this disease. Data demonstrated that the incidence of cancer is increasing, partly because of the fact that the age of our citizenry is increasing. Clearly, cancer strikes more frequently in the older age groups. However, a primary cause for the increased incidence is the sharp increase in lung cancer, probably attributable to a small extent to air pollution in certain environments in our country, but especially to the "self-pollution" of cigarette smoking. The panel estimated that if Americans stopped smoking cigarettes, this alone would eliminate 15% of all cancer deaths in this country within several decades.

Although we do not understand the basic nature of the neoplastic transformation, we know a great deal more about the disease today than we did 50 years ago. In 1930, the medical cure rate for those afflicted with cancer was about one case in five. Today, approximately one in three is cured, and the panel estimated that this could be improved to almost one in two simply by better application of the knowledge which exists today. Certain specific types of tumors that were 100% fatal prior to 1960 can now be cured in as many as 70% of the cases.

Cancer: Yesterday

In all likelihood, all multicellular organisms are afflicted, or have the potential to be afflicted, by the disease we call cancer. Paleopathologists have demonstrated that neoplastic lesions occurred in dinosaur bones long before the advent of *Homo sapiens.* In view of the numerous reports of both spontaneous and induced neoplasms in both plants and animals, vertebrates as well as invertebrates, it is quite probable that cancer has been with us for much of the evolutionary period of life on earth. Ancient Egyptians knew of the existence of cancer in the human patient, and in one papyrus a glyph clearly refers to a clinical tumor (Figure 1). In addition, autopsies of mummies have shown the existence of bone tumors and the probability of other neoplastic processes.

By the era of Hippocrates in the fourth century B.C., many types of neoplasms were clinically recognized and described, such as cancer of the stomach or uterus. Hippocrates coined the term *carcinoma,* which referred to

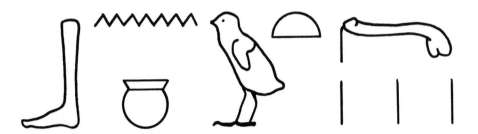

Figure 1: The symbol for "tumor' referring to the surgical treatment of cancer in the hieroglyphics of the Edwin Smith papyrus dating back to more than 1,600 years B.C. The reader is referred to Breasted's translation of the document for further information.

tumors that spread and destroyed the patient. This was in contrast to the group he termed *carcinos,* which included benign tumors, hemorrhoids, and other chronic ulcerations. Almost 600 years later, Galen distinguished "tumors according to nature," such as enlargement of the breast with normal female maturation; "tumors exceeding nature," which included the bony proliferation occurring during the reuniting of a fraction; and "tumors contrary to nature," which today we may define as neoplastic growths. This distinction, proposed some 1800 years ago, is still reasonably correct. Galen also suggested the similarity between a crab and the disease we know today as cancer. Since the latter term is derived from the Latin and carcinoma from the Greek, it is likely that Galen was following in Hippocrates' footsteps.

It was not until the nineteenth century, however, that physicians and scientists began to study cancer systematically and intensively. The anatomist, Bichat, extended the principles of Galen, which had reigned supreme for more than 1,600 years. Bichat described the anatomy of many neoplasms in the human and suggested that cancer was an "accidental formation" of tissue built up in the same manner as any other portion of the organism. Some 17 years later, Johannes Müller extended the findings of Bichat by utilizing the microscope. Although the cellular theory was just being formulated during this period, Müller independently demonstrated that cancer tissue was made up of cells. At this time little was known about cell division, and Pasteur and others had not yet clearly demonstrated the doctrine *omnis cellula e cellula,* i.e., every cell from a cell.

A student of Müller, Rudolf Virchow, dramatically extended our descriptive knowledge of cancer, and, although he proposed a number of theories that were later disproven, he was the first to point out a relationship between chronic irritation and some cancers.

Early in this rapid advance of our knowledge of cancer, two possible pathogenetic bases for the origin of cancer were proposed — that normal cells are converted to cancer cells, or that cancer cells exist from embryonic life but do not express themselves until later in the organism's existence. Müller supported the latter concept, as did Julius Cohnheim at a later period when, in 1877, he advanced the "embryonal rest theory" of cancer. On the other hand, many pathologists such as Laënnec argued that a number of cancers resemble the normal tissues of the body and that "there are as many varieties of these as there are kinds of normal tissues," although Laënnec recognized that a number of tumors bore no direct resemblance to any normal tissue found in the adult organism. Laënnec's studies supported the cellular theory (vide supra) and actually added to it the words *ejusdem naturae* which, combined with the original statement, may be translated as "every cell arises from a cell *of the same kind."*

Another major advance during this period was the demonstration by Waldeyer that metastases were the result of cell emboli. In addition, he was able to show that cells infiltrated from primary cancers into blood and lymphatic vessels.

After major advances had been made in the knowledge of the biology of human neoplasia, experimental oncology emerged as a separate area of knowledge. Experimental tumor transplantation was initiated shortly after the middle of the nineteenth century, and by 1900 some animal neoplasms had been carried through many generations of grafts with few alterations in the microscopic appearance of the neoplasms. The history of studies on the etiology of cancer is fascinating and is dealt with briefly later as part of our discussion of carcinogenesis.

Obviously the experimentalist needs a hypothesis from which he or she formulates and performs experimental investigations. During the nineteenth century, many hypotheses of the origin and development of cancer were presented. In general, however, one may place these into three categories, as follows:

1. The irritation hypothesis
2. The embryonal hypothesis
3. The parasitic hypothesis

Into the first of these could be placed what little was known at that time of the effects of chemical agents, mostly crude, and of radiation in the genesis of cancer. The relationships of some ulcerations, both internal and external, to cancer appeared to support and strengthen this hypothesis. Scar cancers and those occurring after both acute and chronic injury were also cited in support of the irritation hypothesis.

Perhaps the most common example of cancer in support of the embryonal hypothesis is the nevus or common mole of the skin. In most instances these are present from birth, and an extremely tiny percentage of such structures will become cancerous. Many neoplasms of embryonic tissue appearance, such as the teratoma occurring in the adult, would also tend to support this type of hypothesis.

In view of the rapid advances made in our understanding of infectious disease during the last century by Pasteur and numerous others, it is quite understandable that physicians and scientists searched for an infectious origin of cancer. Several reports occurred at the end of the nineteenth century, including that of Doven, who described a bacterium, *Micrococcus neoformans,* which he isolated from several neoplasms and believed to be the cause of all types of cancer. As it turned out, this organism was merely a common staphylococcus. It was not until the twentieth century that this hypothesis became scientifically sound. Even in this century, more than 50 years were to pass before proper scientific recognition was given to the parasitic hypothesis.

Cancer: Today

Cancer has risen from the eighth most common cause of death in the United States in 1900 to the second most common cause of death in 1972, second only to disease of the cardiovascular system. The American Cancer Society has estimated that 345,000 persons died of cancer in the United States in 1972. In all likelihood, this figure will exceed 350,000 in 1978. Except for cancer of the skin, which is the most common and also the most curable of human cancers, 75% of all malignancies in human beings occur in only 10 anatomic sites; these are colon and rectum, breast, lung and bronchus, prostate, uterus, lymph organs, bladder, stomach, blood, and pancreas. In the male the most common site of cancer (other than skin) is the lung and accounts for 22% of cancer in the 1970s; one-third of all deaths from cancer in males result from neoplasms of the lung. The second most common site of incidence is the prostate, but this is only fifth in cause of death and accounts for less than 10% of cancer deaths in the male. In the female, cancer of the breast accounts for 27% of the cases of neoplasia and one-fifth of the deaths from this disease. If males and females are considered together, then the leading types of neoplasms (still excepting skin), accounting for approximately 15% of all cancers, are those of the colon and rectum, followed by breast and lung, with an incidence of 13.6% and 13.3%, respectively.

The age-specific incidence of cancer, when one considers all sites combined, shows that males have a higher incidence than females. The age-specific incidence of frequent sites for males and females is seen in Figure 2. These data are taken from the work of Cutler and his associates. Unfortunately, the data seen in Figure 2 do not tell the whole story. Physicians have been aware for many years that numerous cases of cancer are never diagnosed. While some have argued that the marked increase in the incidence of cancer reported in the human is due to better methods of diagnosis (vide infra), this cannot account for all of the increase seen in this disease. The failure to diagnose cancer is not only related to the lack of contact of the individual with the physician but also to the frequency of the interaction of the patient with the best methods for cancer diagnosis found only in modern hospitals. As the number of hospital admissions increases, the likelihood of an undiagnosed or incorrectly diagnosed case of cancer decreases dramatically. Thus, as medical care for the U.S. population increases in its efficiency and availability, it is quite likely that the patient who seeks medical advice and yet has undiagnosed cancer will become a rarity in our society.

Trends in Cancer Incidence and Mortality

Changes in the incidence of various types of human neoplasms are really the subject of epidemiologic studies. One of the best known examples in this country is the decreasing incidence of cancer of the stomach, in contrast to an increasing incidence of cancer of the lung over the past 25 years. The survival rates of patients with cancer have been increasing, but with a rather interesting pattern. As can be seen in Table 1, the increase in survival rate for many neoplasms was quite significant between the 1940s and the 1950s.

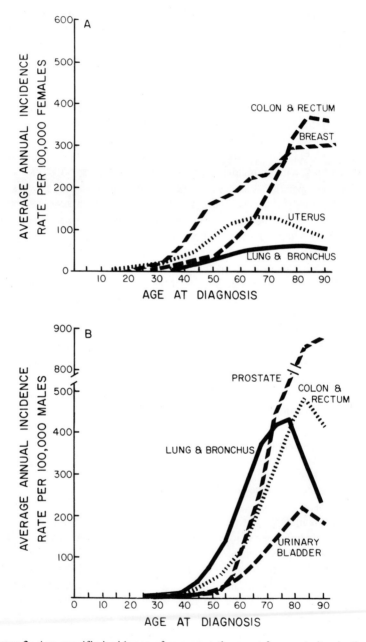

Figure 2: Age-specific incidence of cancer at the most frequent sites in the human. A, females; B, males (After Cutler.)

Table 1. Trend in 5-Year Survival Rates for Cancers[a] Diagnosed in 1940-1969

Primary site	% of all Cancers[b]	5-year relative survival rates (%)[c] according to calendar period of diagnosis			
		1940-49	1950-59	1960-64	1965-69
Breast (females)[d]	13.9	53	60	62	64
Lung	13.1	4	8	9	9
Colon	10.4	32	44	44	45
Prostate[d]	7.9	37	47	52	56
Rectum	4.6	29	40	37	41
Bladder[d]	4.6	42	55	56	60
Corpus[d]	3.8	61	71	73	74
Stomach	3.3	9	12	12	12
Pancreas	3.1	1	1	1	2
Cervix (invasive)	2.7	47	59	57	56
Ovary	2.6	25	29	33	32
Kidney[d]	1.8	26	34	36	41
Brain	1.6	24	25	24	29
Melanoma (skin)[d]	1.5	41	56	62	67
Larynx[d]	1.4	41	56	54	61
Thyroid[d]	1.3	64	80	83	84
Gall bladder	1.0	3	6	8	8
Pharynx	1.0	18	22	24	23
Chronic leukemia[d]	1.4	15	23	27	30
Acute leukemia[d]	1.2	0	1	2	3
Hodgkin's disease	1.1	25	34	42	54
Multiple myeloma[d]	1.1	7	7	11	16
Lymphosarcoma[d]	1.0	23	28	31	32
Leukemia in children:					
All types[d]	e	0	1	4	6
Acute lymphocytic[d]	e	0	0	4	6

[a]Data for white patients only. Data on nonmelanotic skin cancer are not included in this table.

[b]Based on Third National Cancer Survey, 1969-1971.

[c]The relative survival rate adjusts for normal mortality expectation. Thus, meaningful comparisons can be made of survival among patient groups that differ in race, sex, and age.

[d]Continued improvement in survival through 1965-1969.

[e]Included in percentages given above [From Cutler et al., *New Eng. J. Med.* 293 (1975): 122.]

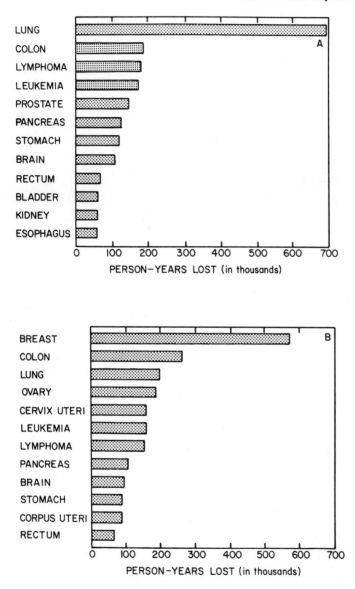

Figure 3: Total and productive years of life lost due to cancer mortality in 1968. A, person-years lost from the leading types of cancer in males; B, person-years lost from the leading types of cancer in females; C, work-years lost from the leading types of cancer in males; D, work-years lost from the leading types of cancer in females. (After Murray and Axtell.)

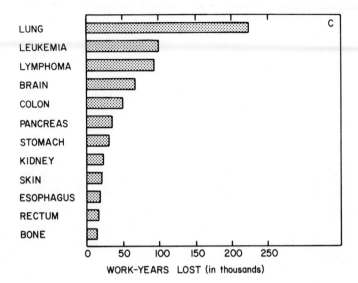

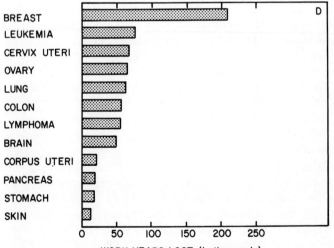

Since 1959 the survival rate has not increased nearly as dramatically. The improvements noted are due to a number of factors, such as:

1. An increase in the proportion of cancers diagnosed at a controllable stage of development resulting from improvements in diagnostic techniques

2. Improvements in surgical and supportive techniques, including the control of infectious disease complicating cancer

3. Improvements in radiotherapy, endocrine therapy, and chemotherapy.

While considerable publicity has been given to the relative leveling off in survival rate for most major neoplasms, it is clear that there is still a steady, albeit slow improvement in the survival rate for virtually all types of neoplasms in the human being. For the first part of the present decade, the trends indicate a continued small but significant increase in survival rates for the types of cancers listed in Table 1.

What is perhaps more significant, and certainly more important to society, is the number of years of life lost because of cancer mortality. If one assumes that the most productive period of a person's life is between the ages of 20 and 65, one can compute the work-years lost during this age interval. From such calculations it is of interest that the person-years lost for females are somewhat higher than for males, despite the greater number of cancer deaths among men. This is a reflection of cancer deaths among women at somewhat younger ages than men and of the longer life expectancy among women than among men for any given age.

The significance of the statistics on deaths resulting from cancer at major sites can be seen from the fact that lung cancer in males in 1968 was three times greater in the person-years lost than its closest competitor, cancer of the colon (Figure 3). Even carcinoma of the breast in the female accounted for only twice the loss of person-years compared with its nearest competitor, cancer of the colon. If one calculates work-years lost on the same basis, then cancer of the lung is not so fearsome and is only twice as serious as its nearest competitor, now leukemia and lymphomas. Likewise, cancer of the breast is about 2-1/2 times as damaging with respect to work-years lost as is leukemia.

Thus the statistics on cancer incidence and cancer mortality are important in our consideration of the impact of this disease on our society. Obviously these figures cannot take into account the morbidity and suffering, both mental and physical, caused by this disease. However, they point out interesting differences in the effects of this disease on males and females and which types of neoplasms are most common in our society and also in other countries. In our later considerations of the epidemiology of cancer we will break down these statistics further in attempting to find explanations for the various incidences of specific neoplasms.

References

F. W. Bauer, S. L. Robbins and J. W. Berg. An autopsy study of cancer patients. II. Hospitalization and accuracy of diagnoses (1955 to 1965) Boston City Hospital. *J. Am. Med. Assoc.* 223 (1973): 299.

W. R. Bett. Historical aspects of cancer. In *Cancer,* Vol. 1 (R. W. Raven, ed.). Butterworth, London, 1957, p. 1.

M. F. X. Bichat. *Anatomie Generale.* Brosson, Gabon and Cie, Paris, 1821.

J. H. Breasted. *The Edwin Smith Surgical Papyrus,* Vol. 1. University of Chicago Press, 1930, pp. 367, 403.

Cancer Facts and Figures. American Cancer Society, 1977.

J. Cohnheim. *Vorlesungen über allgemeine Pathologie.* A. Hirschwald, Berlin, 1877.

S. J. Cutler, M. H. Myers and S. B. Green. Trends in survival rates of patients with cancer. *New Eng. J. Med.* 293 (1975): 122.

S. J. Cutler, J. Scotto, S. S. Devesa and R. R. Connelly. Third National Cancer Survey — An Overview of Available Information. *J. Natl. Cancer Inst.* 53 (1974): 1565.

D. L. Levin, S. S. Devesa, J. D. Godwin and D. T. Silverman. *Cancer Rates and Risks* (2nd ed.). U.S. Department of Health, Education and Welfare, Washington, D.C., 1974.

J. Müller. *Ueber den feineren Bau und die Formen der krankhaften Geschwülste.* Riemer, Berlin, 1838.

J. L. Murray and L. M. Axtell. Impact of cancer: Years of life lost due to cancer mortality. *J. Natl. Cancer Inst.* 52 (1974): 3.

C. Oberling. *The Riddle of Cancer.* Yale University Press, New Haven, 1952.

Report of the National Panel of Consultants on the Conquest of Cancer. U.S. Government Printing Office, Washington, D. C., 1971.

H. Seidman, E. Silverberg, and A. I. Holleb. *Cancer Statistics,* 1976. A comparison of white and black populations. *Ca* 26 (1976): 2.

E. Silverberg and A. I. Holleb. Major Trends in Cancer: 25 Year Survey. *Ca* 25 (1975): 2.

R. Virchow. *Die krankhaften Geschwülste.* A. Hirschwald, Berlin, 1863.

H. W. G. Waldeyer. *Arch. Pathol. Anat. Physiol.* (Virchow's) 55 (1872): 67.

2

The Language of Oncology

The Definition of Neoplasia

As an illustration of the enigma that cancer has presented to physicians and scientists over the years, it was not until the 1920s that meaningful attempts were made to present a definition of cancer. In the ensuing half century a number of definitions of this biological phenomenon have been proposed, mostly by physicians and scientists but more recently also by laymen writing for the scientific press. Some definitions have been rather extensive and detailed, usually reflecting the author's basic experience and research interests; others have been of a more general character. To confuse the field somewhat further, clinicians, scientists, and laymen have used such terms as *cancer, neoplasm, tumor,* and *malignancy* as if such terms were synonymous in every way. Such is not the case. In this text we utilize the terms *neoplasm* and *neoplasia* as the names of the basic disease process defined below. *Cancer* has today become a layman's term which is utilized almost exclusively to indicate a process which has the biological characteristics of a malignant neoplasm (vide infra). The term *malignancy* should also be limited to references to malignant neoplasms. Perhaps the greatest confusion is caused by the use of the word *tumor.* Since the Graeco-Roman era of mankind's understanding of disease, tumor has been used to denote simply a readily defined mass of tissue usually distinctive from normal physiological growth. Thus a scar, a healing bone or callus, "proud flesh," a granuloma, a chronic abscess, or a parasitic mass are all tumors, but are not neoplasms. Part of this confusion arises from the fact that several English pathologists have employed the term *tumour* synonymously with neoplasia. In this text, however, we do not use this latter terminology.

15

While most of the definitions of neoplasia that have been proposed have generally common themes, we utilize the definition proposed by the pathologist, James Ewing. The following is Ewing's definition, slightly modified:

A neoplasm is a relatively autonomous growth of tissue.

This definition encompasses several things. The first of these is *relative autonomy*. Autonomy indicates that a cancer is not subject to the "rules and regulations" that govern the individual cells and the overall cell interactions of the functional organism. The adjective, *relative,* modifies this term to indicate that neoplasms are not completely autonomous. In many instances the autonomy that a neoplasm possesses may be quite subtle and relative only to the tissue from which it arose. However, it should be emphasized that this phrase, *relative autonomy,* is by far the most important aspect of the definition and sets off a particular cell type as being neoplastic in the general sense. Relative autonomy is used here in the biological sense, but it is anticipated that one day we will understand it in the molecular sense; when we do, we will probably understand the mechanisms of the malignant process itself.

The second essential component of the definition is the term *growth.* Growth here may indicate the rate of cell division or the rate of intracellular processes involved in the synthesis of macromolecules for use within the cell or for excretion by the cell. The actual *rate* of growth may be extremely low, differing little from that in the normal counterpart of the neoplasm; or, in the most serious cases, the rate may be extremely rapid, approaching that of the growth rate of embryonic tissue. In some instances, as with neoplasms of the small intestine or certain chronic leukemias (vide infra), the rate of growth of the neoplastic cell may be less than that of its normal counterpart. Obviously, if the cells of a neoplasm do not proliferate to a point where the tumor is grossly or histologically recognizable, it is practically impossible to designate the cellular population as a tumor or a neoplasm. Thus, enhanced cell replication, in fact, becomes a part of the operational definition of neoplasia, although from the experiments of Fisher and Fisher we recognize that neoplastic cells may exist for a lifetime in the host without ever undergoing demonstrable cell division. These experiments are discussed in Chapter 8.

Finally, the third component of the definition is the term *tissue.* This term requires that, at our present state of knowledge, cancer or neoplasia can be defined only in a multicellular organism. By this definition, unicellular organisms are free of this disease. Thus, in fact, cancer becomes "the curse of evolution."

The definition of neoplasia proposed by Ewing in the mid-1930s was that of a pathologist knowledgeable in the biology of cancer expressed in vivo. Today, the in vivo system is still the basic reference for our definition of the neoplastic cell. On the other hand, with the recent advances of carcinogenesis in vitro, characteristics of the cancer cell growing in tissue culture have been described. Although it is not yet possible to define the malignant cell in vitro without reference to its behavior in vivo, the ultimate goal of experimental oncology is to elucidate the molecular definition of the cancer cell regardless of its environment.

Types of Growth (Plasias)

Hyperplasia

The term *hyperplasia* has been used to denote an increase in cell number. As you may already have learned, *hypertrophy* indicates an increase in cell size but not in cell number. Although many neoplasms are characterized by hyperplasia, many normal tissues are also characterized by a dramatic increase in cell number. Embryonic tissue has perhaps the fastest rate of hyperplasia, but some adult tissues, especially those involved in certain metabolic functions such as the crypt cells of the small intestine, cells of the bone marrow, and, to a lesser extent, the cells of the basal layer of the skin, are normally hyperplastic. In reactions such as wound healing and callus formation, hyperplasia is a normal process. Thus, hyperplasia may occur in cancer but is not a unique characteristic or even an absolute requirement of neoplasia.

Metaplasia

Metaplasia is a reversible process in which one adult cell type in a specific organ or organ structure is replaced by another adult cell type. In most instances the secondary or replacing cell type is not normally seen in the particular region in which the metaplasia occurs. Metaplasia may be either epithelial or mesenchymal.

The most common example of *epithelial metaplasia* is in the change of columnar or pseudostratified columnar epithelium of the respiratory tract to squamous epithelium. This phenomenon is known as squamous metaplasia and may result from numerous stimuli, among which are chronic irritation and inflammation. The mechanism of metaplasia in epithelial cells is not the direct transformation of one cell type to another, but rather a redirection of the differentiation of a stem cell. In the respiratory tract the stem cell normally gives rise to pseudostratified columnar epithelium, but in the presence of certain stimuli it may differentiate into squamous epithelium. It would appear that vitamin A may be associated with such squamous metaplasia, since animals that are deficient in this vitamin show extensive squamous metaplasia of mucous columnar epithelium, whereas treatment with vitamin A may reverse the squamous metaplasia.

The appearance of mucous columnar epithelium and its conversion to squamous epithelium by vitamin A deficiency with its reversal back to its original form when vitamin A is again added to the diet is shown schematically in Figure 4. The mechanism of this metaplasia appears to be a redifferentiation of certain stem cells (shown as small black nuclei along the basement membrane) of each of the epithelia seen in Figure 4. Since these epithelial cells are constantly being replaced by progeny of the stem cells, in the absence of vitamin A or some other chronic stimulus as yet undefined, the differentiation of the stem cell may be redirected to the more primitive squamous epithelium. In the presence of vitamin A or some other unknown environmental factor, normal differentiation of the stem cell may recur. A further discussion of the effect of vitamin A on carcinogenesis may be found in Chapter 7.

Mesenchymal metaplasia may be the result of stem cell differentiation but may also occur by "transformation" of one cell type into another. In cell culture, such conversion of one cell type to another can occur in the absence of cell division.

Anaplasia and Dysplasia

Robbins defines *dysplasia* as "an alteration in adult cells characterized by variation in their size, shape and organization." This term has confused a number of individuals, especially when it is contrasted with the term *anaplasia,* which is characterized at two different biological levels by alterations in intracellular macromolecular syntheses and intercellular relationships and associations as described below. Dysplasia is a more common term used by pathologists and, in general, would appear to refer primarily to the arrangement and size of cells.

Positional or *organizational anaplasia* refers to the interrelationship of cells in a specific tissue. Normally there are distinct histologic patterns in tissues. When positional anaplasia occurs, these distinct patterns are altered, in that either cell organelles are arranged randomly with respect to one another in adjacent cells, or cells are disarranged with respect to one another.

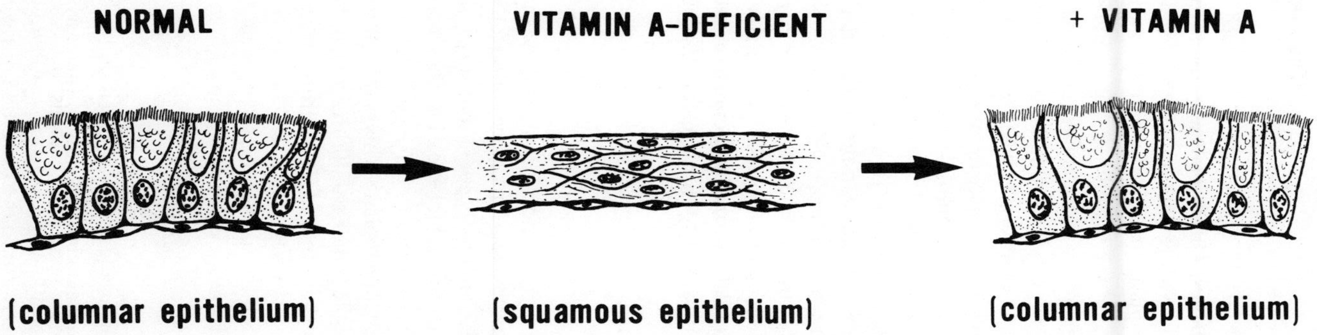

NORMAL

(columnar epithelium)

VITAMIN A-DEFICIENT

(squamous epithelium)

+ VITAMIN A

(columnar epithelium)

Figure 4: Artist's representation of the morphologic changes occurring in the metaplasia of ciliated columnar epithelium to squamous epithelium in vitamin A-deficient animals and the subsequent redifferentiation of the squamous epithelium to columnar epithelium in the presence of vitamin A.

Cytologic anaplasia is largely a function of increased or altered nucleic acid synthesis in growing tissues. This term usually refers to the staining characteristics of cells, especially with respect to basophilia and the nuclear/cytoplasmic ratio. Cytologic anaplasia may also be a function of the ploidy of the cell; it is seen normally in the placenta, a callus, and occasionally in wound healing. Cytologic anaplasia is extremely important in the cytologic diagnosis of malignancy. However, it should be emphasized that since normal tissues may exhibit cytologic anaplasia as well as positional anaplasia, this phenomenon is not an absolute characteristic of malignancy.

In Figure 5 may be seen a conceptual drawing of both positional and cytologic anaplasia. The artist's conception demonstrates that in positional anaplasia there is an alteration in the distribution in space of cell organelles within a specific tissue or epithelium, or in the spatial relationship of one cell or group of cells to another within a tissue. Cytologic anaplasia is shown as a distortion of cellular architecture as compared with the normal cell type and is characterized by intensified staining (denoted by the darkened nuclei) of the nucleus and cytoplasm of the cell. The reader should be aware, however, that in many neoplasms both positional and cytologic anaplasia occur simultaneously.

Neoplasia

We have already defined a neoplasm and, thus, neoplasia as a relatively autonomous growth of tissue. In the next sections, as we consider the classification of neoplasms, certain contradictions may become apparent. It should be emphasized that all neoplasms, regardless of their biological behavior, come under this classification. In this sense the terms *cancer* and *malignancy* may occasionally be used synonymously with neoplasm or neoplasia. This may be done without reference to the biological behavior of the tumor, and for this reason the student must be on guard to insure that the actual meaning of these terms is clear when they are used.

The Classification of Neoplasms

Behavioristic (Biological) Classification

Since our definition of neoplasia is presently based on the biological behavior of tumors, it is proper to make a classification on the basis of such behavior. However, it should be noted in making this classification that all neoplasms which we are considering conform to the definition of Ewing. As we shall see, the distinction between benign and malignant neoplasms in the behavioristic classification has considerable usefulness in determining the prognosis

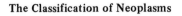

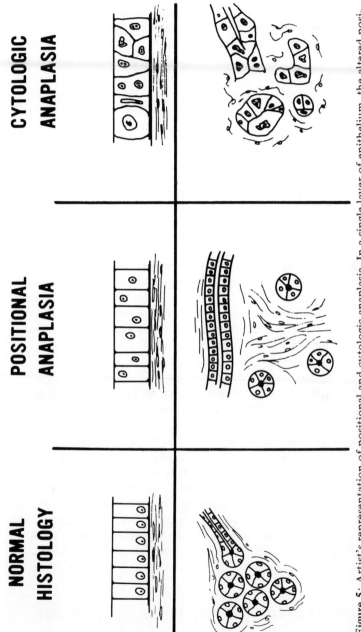

Figure 5: Artist's representation of positional and cytologic anaplasia. In a single layer of epithelium, the altered position of nuclei in relation to one another in adjacent cells is depicted as well as the altered position of ducts and glands in a specific representative structure. Cytologic anaplasia is noted by the marked variation in nuclear size and staining characteristics, nucleolar size, and nuclear-cytoplasmic ratio.

of cancer in a specific patient, but is of little use to the scientist who is studying the mechanisms of neoplasia at the molecular level.

The principal behavioristic characteristics of benign and malignant neoplasms are as follows:

Benign	Malignant
1. Encapsulated	Non-encapsulated
2. Noninvasive	Invasive
3. Highly differentiated	Poorly differentiated
4. Rare mitoses	Mitoses relatively common
5. Slow growth	Rapid growth
6. Little or no anaplasia	Anaplastic to varying degrees
7. No metastases	Metastases

As can be seen, the majority of differences between benign and malignant neoplasms are relative. The critical difference between the two types is point 7, in that benign neoplasms by definition do not metastasize, whereas malignant tumors have this capability. A metastasis is defined as the secondary growth of a neoplasm, originating from the primary tumor and growing within the host organism in a location distant from the initial site of neoplastic growth. As we shall see in Chapter 8, there are various routes and mechanisms of metastases for malignant neoplasms.

While there is little doubt from the literature that most pathologists and students of oncology define a malignant neoplasm by its ability to metastasize, the artificiality of this distinction from the viewpoint of the natural history of neoplasia will soon become evident to the student. The fact that a number of benign neoplasms may at some time during their natural history take on the behavior of a malignant neoplasm is well known. This phenomenon, which we shall later discuss under the heading "Progression of Neoplasms," was emphasized to a large degree by Foulds and his students, even to the point that this famous oncologist considered the behavioristic distinction between benign and malignant neoplasms to be essentially nonexistent. However, the fact remains that students of oncology have made the distinction between benign and malignant neoplasms that we have presented here. The significance of this technical distinction between the two has recently assumed greater importance in relation to carcinogen testing and the potential carcinogenicity to humans of chemicals in our environment (see Chapter 5).

The Histogenetic Classification of Neoplasms

Although the behavioristic classification is one of the most commonly accepted segments of the nomenclature of neoplasms, the most important principle in the classification of neoplasms is their grouping according to the type of tissue from which the neoplasm has arisen (Table 2). Ritchie distinguishes groups of neoplasms on the basis of their histogenetic origin as follows:

1. Neoplasms of epithelium

2. Neoplasms of connective tissue

3. Neoplasms of the hematopoietic and immune systems

4. Neoplasms of the nervous system

5. Neoplasms of multiple histogenetic celluclar origin

6. Miscellaneous neoplasms

This classification has considerable usefulness in itself, especially when considered with other aspects of the lesions, both from the diagnostic and the biological viewpoint. For example, it is very important to determine the region, organ, or tissue from which the neoplasm arose. In addition, other descriptive terms are often utilized in classifying or diagnosing a specific neoplasm. Such descriptive terms as papillary, cystic, follicular, etc., may relate to various histologic types of neoplasms of epithelial origin. In addition, some neoplasms have been named according to the individual first describing the tumor; examples are Ewing's tumor of bone, Hodgkin's disease of lumph tissue, and Wilms' tumor of the kidney.

Nomenclature of Neoplasms and
Its Embryologic Basis

In order to discuss the phenomenon of neoplasia, it is important that certain aspects of currently accepted nomenclature be understood. It should be noted, however, that there is no one system of nomenclature of neoplasms used worldwide. In this country nomenclature has revolved around the use of the suffix, *-oma,* which literally means "tumor." With few exceptions,

Table 2. Examples of Neoplasms Based on the Histogenetic Classification[a]

Tissue of Origin	Benign	Malignant
1. Epithelial neoplasms		
Epidermis	Epidermal papilloma	Epidermal carcinoma
Stomach	Gastric polyp	Gastric carcinoma
Biliary tree	Cholangioma	Cholangiocarcinoma
Adrenal cortex	Adrenocortical adenoma	Adrenocortical carcinoma
2. Connective tissue neoplasms		
Fibrous tissue	Fibroma	Fibrosarcoma
Cartilage	Chondroma	Chondrosarcoma
Bone	Osteoma	Osteogenic sarcoma
Fat	Lipoma	Liposarcoma
Smooth muscle	Leiomyoma	Leiomyosarcoma
Skeletal muscle	Rhabdomyoma	Rhabdomyosarcoma
3. Neoplasms of the hemopoietic and immune systems		
Lymphoid tissue	Brill-Symmer's disease	Lymphosarcoma (lymphoma)
		Lymphatic leukemia
		Reticulum-cell sarcoma
		Hodgkin's disease
Thymus	Thymoma	Thymoma
Granulocytes		Myelogenous leukemia
Erythrocytes	Polycythemia vera	Erythroleukemia
Plasma cells		Multiple myeloma
4. Neoplasms of the nervous system		
Glia	Astrocytoma	Glioblastoma multiforme
	Oligodendroglioma	
Meninges	Meningioma	Meningeal sarcoma
Neurons	Ganglioneuroma	Neuroblastoma
Adrenal medulla	Phaeochromocytoma	
5. Neoplasms of multiple tissues		
Breast	Fibroadenoma	Cystosarcoma phylloides
Kidney		Wilms' tumor
Ovary, testis, etc.	Dermoid (benign teratoma)	Malignant teratoma
6. Miscellaneous neoplasms		
Melanocytes	Nevus	Melanoma
Placenta	Hydatiform mole	Chorionepithelioma
Ovary	Granulosa cell tumor	Granulosa cell tumor
	Cystadenoma	Cystadenocarcinoma
Testis		Seminoma

[a]After Ritchie, 1962.

words with this suffix do refer to neoplasms. An exception is the term, *granuloma,* which is a nonneoplastic tumor of inflammatory tissue.

In the behavioristic classification, benign tumors may be named with a prefix that refers to the tissue from which the neoplasm arose and with the suffix -oma. For example, a benign neoplasm of fibrous tissue is called a fibroma; a benign neoplasm of cartilage, a chondroma; a benign neoplasm of glandular tissue, an adenoma, etc. When one considers the malignant tumors, however, some other aspects of classification enter in. Malignant neoplasms are divided into two general categories, depending on their embryologic origin. Figure 6 outlines some of the steps in the early development of a fertilized egg of higher vertebrate animals. After fertilization the egg divides a number of times giving rise to 2-, 4-, 8-, 16-, 32-, etc., cell stages which form a small spherical structure, termed the blastula, which has a central cavity. Continued development of this structure to the gastrula involves an invagination of the cells of one part of the surface giving rise to a small "ball within a ball," as diagrammed in cross section in Figure 6. At this stage it is possible for the embryologist to distinguish three different layers of cells. The outer-most layer is termed the ectoderm and develops to give rise to the skin and its associated structures in the adult. The layer of invaginated cells is termed the endoderm and ultimately gives rise to the gastrointestinal tract and its associated structures. In between these two layers a mass of cells forms in the gastrula which is termed the mesoderm, giving rise in the adult to supporting structures such as bone, fat, muscle, blood, etc. As can be seen from the figure, a malignant neoplasm arising from derivatives of the mesodermal (mesenchymal) embryonic germ layer is termed a *sarcoma.* If the neoplasm arises from tissues derived from embryonic ecto- or endoderm, the term *carcinoma* applies to malignant neoplasms of such tissues. Thus the terms adenocarcinoma of the stomach, the pancreas, or the breast are appropriate nomenclature for malignant neoplasms of the epithelium of these organs. On the other hand, a liposarcoma may arise from the fat tissue of the breast, a chondrosarcoma from cartilage of the ribs, or an osteogenic sarcoma from the bony rib itself.

Several terms do not fit strictly into this type of nomenclature. The suffix *blastoma* is used to denote certain types of neoplasms to indicate that the tissue has a primitive appearance that resembles embryologic structures. Examples of this are the neuroblastoma and the myoblastoma. In other examples of nomenclature the terminology is rather confusing. A highly malignant tumor that has the appearance of both a carcinoma and a sarcoma is termed a *carcinosarcoma.* This would indicate that the neoplasm was derived from two germ layers. Another condition, the "mixed" tumor of the salivary

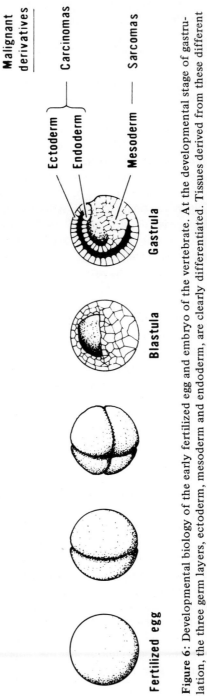

Figure 6: Developmental biology of the early fertilized egg and embryo of the vertebrate. At the developmental stage of gastrulation, the three germ layers, ectoderm, mesoderm and endoderm, are clearly differentiated. Tissues derived from these different layers may give rise to malignant neoplasms with the terminology based on their germ layer of derivation. See text for further details.

gland, which is definitely not a carcinosarcoma, was also thought to have this embryonic derivation. It is now felt that the mixed tumor is probably a low-grade carcinoma, and the term carcinosarcoma should be reserved only for highly malignant, quite primitive tumors with the histologic characteristics mentioned above.

The most common neoplasm of multiple-tissue origin is known as the *teratoma,* which is a tumor derived from all three germ layers. These neoplasms may be either benign or malignant in the behavioristic sense.

Table 2 lists several neoplasms classified according to the behavioristic and histogenetic methods. Although the rules of classification mentioned in this outline are reasonably inclusive, there are some exceptions in the designation of specific neoplasms, as can be seen from the table. For example, the melanoma is not a benign neoplasm but rather a highly malignant tumor of melanocytes. The hepatoma, although the term suggests a benign neoplasm, is, in almost all instances, malignant. As your knowledge of experimental oncology increases, the specific exceptions to the rules will become more familiar.

References

L. V. Ackerman and J. A. delRegato. *Cancer–Diagnosis, Treatment and Prognosis.* Mosby, St. Louis, 1962, p. 77.

J. Bland-Sutton. *Tumors–Innocent and Malignant* (5th ed.). Cassell, London, 1911, p. 8.

D. F. Cappell. *Muir's Textbook of Pathology* (7th ed.). Edward Arnold, London, 1958, p. 224.

J. Ewing. *Neoplastic Disease: A Treatise on Tumors* (4th ed.). Saunders, Philadelphia, 1940.

H. C. Hopps. *Principles of Pathology* (2nd ed.). Appleton-Century-Crofts, New York, 1964, p. 311.

T. H. Maugh, II and J. L. Marx. *Seeds of Destruction–The Science Report on Cancer Research.* Plenum, New York, 1975.

G. L. Montgomery. *Textbook of Pathology.* Williams and Wilkins, Baltimore, 1965, p. 95.

A. C. Ritchie. *The classification, morphology and behavior of tumors.* In *General Pathology* (H. Florey, ed.). Saunders, Philadelphia, 1962, p. 551.

S. L. Robbins. *Pathologic Basis of Disease.* Saunders, Philadelphia, 1974,
     p. 106.
S. L. Robbins. *The Pathologic Basis of Disease.* Saunders, Philadelphia, 1974,
     p. 118.
J. B. Walter and M. S. Israel. *General Pathology* (4th ed.). Churchill Living-
     ston, London, 1974, p. 312.
J. B. Walter and M. S. Israel. *General Pathology* (4th ed.). Churchill Living-
     ston, London, 1974, pp. 314 and 324.

3

The Etiology of Cancer: Chemical and Physical Agents

One of the earliest beginnings of our understanding of carcinogenesis dates back to 1775 and the report by Percival Pott, an astute English surgeon, on the clinical observation of scrotal cancer in adults who had been chimney sweeps during childhood. Doctor Pott, with remarkable insight, ascribed the high incidence of this rather peculiar type of malignancy in this social group as resulting from their childhood occupation and their extensive contact with soot. This association of incompletely oxidized organic molecules and skin cancer was not intensively investigated again until 140 years later, although in the latter part of the nineteenth century and the early twentieth century there was considerable concern about the development of skin cancer in people working in the leather industry and in certain other industries involving heavy exposure to oils and soots.

Before embarking on a discussion of the causation of cancer, it again becomes important to add to our vocabulary. The term *carcinogen* has been generally used by oncologists to indicate an agent that causes cancer. However, as our knowledge of oncology increases, this simplistic definition is not sufficient. Drs. James and Elizabeth Miller have proposed the following definition to include most instances of agents that are carcinogens, while at the same time excluding those agents that do not have a direct action on the cell undergoing the neoplastic transformation.

A *carcinogen* is an agent whose administration to previously untreated animals leads to a statistically significant increased incidence of malignant neoplasms as compared with that in untreated appropriate control animals, whether the control animals have

29

low or high spontaneous incidences of the neoplasms in question. While it would be important to distinguish between agents that produce malignant neoplasms by direct action on the cells that become malignant and those that produce malignancy by indirect actions in the animals, at present it is seldom possible to do so. Some agents, including promoters (Chapter 6) and immune suppressants, can increase the incidence of malignant neoplasms in tissues previously treated with subcarcinogenic doses of carcinogens; such agents should not be termed carcinogens.

Chemical Carcinogenesis

In 1915 the Japanese pathologists Yamagiwa and Ichikawa reported the first production of skin tumors in animals by the application of coal tar to the skin. These investigators applied crude coal tar to the ears of rabbits and produced both benign and, later, malignant epidermal neoplasms. Further studies demonstrated that the skin of mice was also susceptible to the carcinogenic action of organic tars. During the next 15 years extensive attempts were made to determine the nature of the material in the crude tars that caused malignancy. In 1925 Kennaway demonstrated the production of carcinogenic tars from simple organic compounds consisting only of carbon and hydrogen. In the early 1930s several polycyclic hydrocarbons were isolated from active crude tar fractions. In 1930 Kennaway synthesized the compound, 1,2,5,6-dibenzanthracene, a potent polycyclic hydrocarbon carcinogen. The structures of several polycyclic hydrocarbons and other chemical carcinogens are given in Figure 7. Polycyclic hydrocarbons vary in their carcinogenic potency, and the compound, 1,2,3,4-dibenzanthracene, has very little carcinogenic activity. One of the most potent hydrocarbon carcinogens yet described is 3-methylcholanthrene. Numerous studies have been carried out on these compounds in an attempt to determine the exact molecular configuration responsible for carcinogenic potency. With the exception of the designation of certain molecular configurations known as the L and K regions, as well as the fact that most of the hydrocarbons are planar, no dramatic generalizations developed from these early studies. However, planarity of the molecule is not essential to carcinogenicity, since the angular ring of 7,12-dimethylbenz(a)-anthracene, another potent hydrocarbon carcinogen, is approximately $15°$ out of the plane of the rest of the molecule.

In 1935 Sasaki and Yoshida opened up another field of chemical carcinogenesis by demonstrating that the feeding of the azo dye, o-aminoazo-

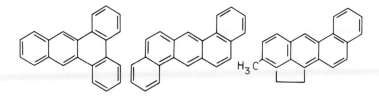

1:2:3:4—dibenzanthracene 1:2:5:6—dibenzanthracene 3—methylchloranthrene

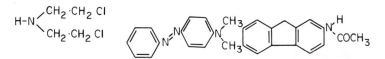

bis(2—chloroethyl)amine 4—dimethylaminoazobenzene 2—acetylaminofluorene

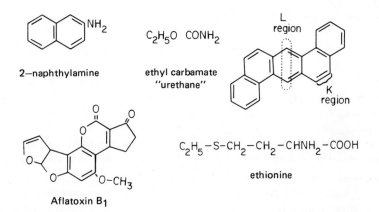

2—naphthylamine

ethyl carbamate "urethane"

C_2H_5O $CONH_2$

L region

K region

$C_2H_5-S-CH_2-CH_2-CHNH_2-COOH$

ethionine

Aflatoxin B$_1$

Figure 7: Chemical structures of several representative chemical carcinogens and their isomers.

toluene, to rats resulted in the development of liver tumors. Kinosita later demonstrated that 4-dimethylaminoazobenzene could also cause the production of neoplasms in the liver. A number of analogs of this compound were also prepared. The interesting correlation arising from these studies was the fact that the amino group of carcinogenic dyes usually had at least one methyl substituent. It should be noted that, unlike the polycyclic hydrocarbons, the azo dyes, in general, did not act at the site of contact of the compound with the organism, but rather in a remote area, the liver. Skin painting with most azo dyes resulted in few or no tumors, and the feeding of polycyclic hydrocarbons except in the neonatal period has generally resulted in no hepatomas. Another important carcinogen that acts at remote sites is 2-acetylaminofluorene, which, though initially prepared as an insecticide, was never used for this purpose. In addition, the amines, beta-naphthylamine and 4-aminobiphenyl, have been shown to be carcinogenic for the urinary bladder in humans. Another remotely acting carcinogen is ethyl carbamate, which appears to be a general "initiating agent" in the mouse (Chapter 6). Ethyl carbamate was used therapeutically in humans before its carcinogenic potency was known. Furthermore, certain cytocidal drugs, such as the nitrogen mustards, which have been used to treat cancer in a number of human patients, have been shown to be potent carcinogens.

In addition to the carcinogenic compounds shown in Figure 7, two other classes of compounds have been shown to be potent carcinogens and to be of potential importance in the genesis of neoplasia in the human being. The dialkylnitrosamines have the general structure $R_1 R_2 - N - N = O$, in which R_1 and R_2 can be any of a variety of alkyl substituents or can be fused to yield a cyclic aliphatic substituent. The simplest nitrosamine, dimethylnitrosamine, is highly carcinogenic for the liver and kidney in rodents and in all other mammals tested. Hepatic toxicity was shown to occur in humans working with dimethylnitrosamine at the time of its earliest industrial use. Subsequently, this source of exposure was eliminated by cessation of the industrial use of nitrosamines as solvents. Recently several investigators have proposed and shown in experimental animals that certain dietary components, especially in the presence of high levels of nitrite, may give rise to nitrosamines in the food or in vivo. This has also been shown to occur by the action of bacterial flora within the intestine.

Another important environmental as well as experimental hepatocarcinogenic agent is aflatoxin B_1. This toxic substance is produced by certain strains of the mold *Aspergillus flavus*. Aflatoxin B_1 is the most potent hepatocarcinogenic agent known and has been shown to be capable of producing neoplasms in rodents, fish, birds, and primates. The material is a potential contaminant of many farm products that are improperly stored for some length of time, e.g., grain, peanuts, etc. It is felt that this compound and related compounds may cause some of the toxic hepatitis and hepatic neoplasia seen in various parts of Africa.

In addition to the various chemicals listed above, certain inorganic compounds have also been shown to possess potent carcinogenic properties. Recent studies have shown that nickel oxides and sulfides are capable of producing muscle tumors in rodents. Beryllium, when given to animals, may produce bone tumors, or if inhaled it is capable of producing pulmonary neoplasms. In humans there is evidence that arsenic, whether through contact or ingestion, may produce cancer of the skin. In rodents, however, this compound does not appear to be carcinogenic.

Although the discovery that polycyclic hydrocarbons could produce cancer indicated that the complete understanding of the nature of neoplasia might be at hand, more than 40 years have elapsed and we still appear to be a long way from such an understanding. The demonstration of the K region suggested a specific relationship of these compounds to some chemical sites. However, the primary metabolites of polycyclic hydrocarbons were found to be hydroxylated derivatives, which usually had little or no carcinogenic activity. Similarly, hydroxylation of the rings of the aromatic amine carcinogens, such as 2-acetylaminofluorene (AAF) and 4-dimethylaminoazobenzene (DAB), usually resulted in a complete loss of activity.

The most significant advance in this field was made by the Millers, who demonstrated that another metabolite of AAF was the N-hydroxy derivative. This derivative was found to be more carcinogenic than its parent compound. N-hydroxy-AAF could also induce neoplasms that the parent compound was unable to induce, such as subcutaneous sarcomas at sites of injection of the N-hydorxy derivative. Furthermore, in animals (such as the guinea pig) that did not possess the enzymatic capacity to convert AAF to its N-hydroxy derivative, cancers could not be produced by feeding the parent compound. These studies strongly supported the suggestion that, at least in the case of AAF, the parent compound was not the direct carcinogen, but rather that certain derivatives were the active components in the induction of neoplasia. These studies paved the way to a study of the activation of carcinogens through their metabolism by cells. Figure 8, taken from a recent review by Weisburger and Williams, illustrates many of the metabolic pathways of carcinogens that lead to more active "proximate" carcinogens. The "ultimate" form of the carcinogen, i.e., the form that actually interacts with cellular constituents to cause the neoplastic transformation, is probably the final product shown in most of the pathways seen in Figure 8. However, in some instances it is still not clear what the ultimate form of a carcinogenic substance is. In other cases there may be more than one ultimate carcinogenic metabolite.

All of these studies taken together demonstrate that many, if not the vast majority of, chemical carcinogens must be metabolized within the cell before they exert their carcinogenic activity. In this respect carcinogenesis becomes a "lethal synthesis" analagous to the earlier studies by Peters, who coined the term with reference to fluoroacetate. Furthermore, this finding ex-

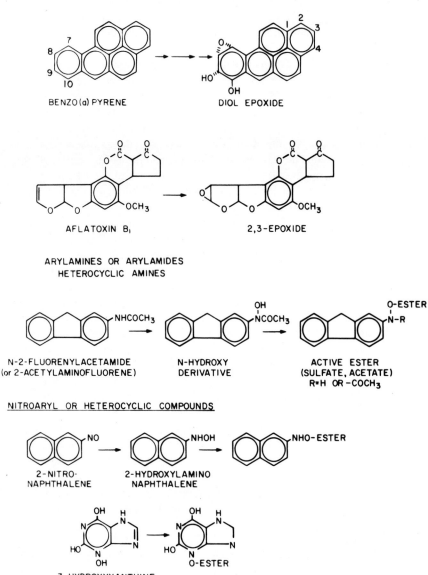

Figure 8: Structures of representative chemical carcinogens and their metabolic derivatives, the proximate and ultimate carcinogenic forms. (After Weisburger and Williams.)

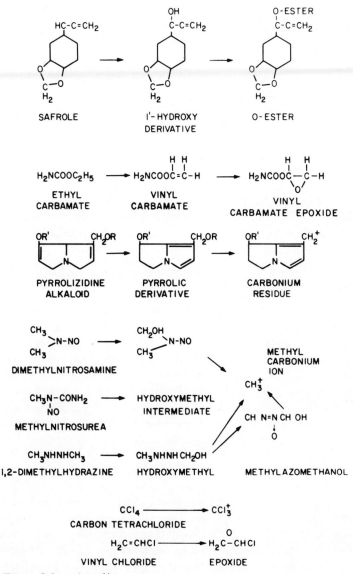

Figure 8 (continued)

plains how a substance that is not carcinogenic for one species may be carcinogenic for another, the result depending on the metabolic capacities present within the species itself. This becomes extremely important for carcinogen testing in whole animals. In tests of the mutagenicity of chemical carcinogens, early studies by the Millers and Szybalski demonstrated that, whereas AAF itself is not mutagenic, one of its metabolites, AAF-N-sulfate, is highly mutagenic for transforming DNA systems. This and other findings led to the mutagenesis assay for chemical carcinogens established by Ames and his associates, which involves the in vitro metabolism of suspected carcinogens by liver microsomal preparations in the presence of a highly mutable strain of bacteria. In this way, if any active metabolite is produced, mutagenesis of the bacteria can occur even if the original compound shows no mutagenic activity. A similar system can be established in vivo but is somewhat more cumbersome.

In 1947 the Millers first demonstrated that during the process of hepatocarcinogenesis azo dyes become covalently bound to proteins of the liver but not to proteins of the resulting neoplasms. Sorof and his associates studied the proteins of liver that bind dyes and demonstrated that azo dye-induced hepatomas did not contain these protein species as judged by electrophoresis and other sensitive methods. Studies with more highly differentiated hepatocellular carcinomas have shown the presence of the dye-binding proteins, but there is still little or no binding of carcinogens that are fed to animals bearing these neoplasms in vivo. These studies led to the original postulation of the "deletion hypothesis" by the Millers, which stated that the binding of carcinogens to proteins led to the loss or deletion of these proteins in the subsequent neoplastic cell. Although this hypothesis has not withstood the test of time in its original form, the reader must recall that it was proposed at a time when we understood very little about the molecular biology of nucleic acids and mutational effects. Since the early studies of the Millers, carcinogens have been found to bind not only to proteins but also to nucleic acids, both DNA and RNA, and possibly to other macromolecular species such as glycogen. The covalent association of carcinogens with lipids has not been adequately studied as yet.

One important question in chemical carcinogenesis obviously is the nature of the critical molecular interaction between the ultimate carcinogen and that component of the cell whose reaction with the carcinogen leads to the neoplastic change. Numerous metabolic studies with labeled carcinogens have investigated the loss of radioactivity from protein, RNA, and DNA, and have shown that label is almost entirely lost from the former two components but is always retained to some small extent by the DNA of cells. These findings have led to the postulation that the interaction critical to the neoplastic transformation is between the ultimate form of the carcinogen and DNA. Other studies have demonstrated that many carcinogens cause damage to DNA which may be repaired by mechanisms very similar to the repair of DNA damaged by ultraviolet light. Many investigators have suggested that if the repair is not accurate, mutations will arise as a result. The mutagenicity of the ultimate carcinogens is a further indication of the importance of the interaction between the carcinogen and DNA, on the assumption that carcinogenesis is the result of mutagenesis. Although the latter is still an assumption, today it is clear that the vast majority of chemical carcinogens either are themselves mutagens or may be converted in the cell to an active mutagen. Thus the majority of such evidence supports the suggestion that chemical carcinogens may exert their effects by a direct interaction of the ultimate form of the carcinogen with cellular DNA itself.

One class of carcinogens has been described that does not conform to any of the concepts related above. This is the group of inert plastics and metals that, upon implantation in rodents, cause sarcomas at the implantation site. There is no generally accepted theory as to the mechanism of this so-called "plastic film" carcinogenesis, but studies by Brand and his associates have suggested that the presence of the film stimulates the production of specific "preneoplastic" clones of cells that ultimately give rise to the sarcomas. It is of interest that multiple perforations or powdering of the plastic implant causes a marked reduction or complete loss of its carcinogenic capabilities. Therefore, the chemical nature of the implant is not the critical factor in its ability to transform normal to neoplastic cells.

Hormonal Induction of Neoplasia

The concept that hormones may be a causative factor(s) in the development of specific types of neoplasms was first pointed out by Beatson, who at the end of the last century suggested a relationship between breast cancer and the ovary. Within the past 30 years such a concept has been reinforced by several experimental systems, and within the past 5 years hormonally induced cancer in humans has become a subject of great significance to our society.

The physiological role of hormones in maintaining the "internal milieu" (Claude Bernard) is now a well-accepted scientific fact. That cancer can result from abnormal production internally or the excessive external administration of hormones represents an interesting pathway of carcinogenesis, since such a phenomenon indicates that the mere derangement of an organism's homeostatic mechanisms may result in the neoplastic transformation. Furth and his associates have been most vocal in their propositions and demonstrations that disruption of the cybernetic relationships between the endocrine glands and the anterior pituitary may result in neoplasia of one or the other of the glands involved. These cybernetic relationships are graphically depicted in Figure 9 for a number of the more common peripheral endocrine-related organs and the pituitary. According to the hypothesis of Furth, break-age of any of the feedback relationships may result in a neoplasm of the glands involved. One of the classical examples is the experimental transplantation of normal ovaries into the spleen of castrated rodents. This results in a break in the pituitary-gonadal hormone feedback loop, since estrogens produced by the ovary are carried by the splenic venous system to the liver where they are metabolized, never entering the general circulation to suppress the pituitary production of gonadotropins. The excessive production of gonadotropins and their constant stimulus to the ovarian fragment in the spleen results ultimately in neoplasia of the ovarian splenic implant. In the reverse direction, neoplasms of the anterior pituitary may be induced by thyroidectomy, presumably by an exaggeration of a negative feedback as

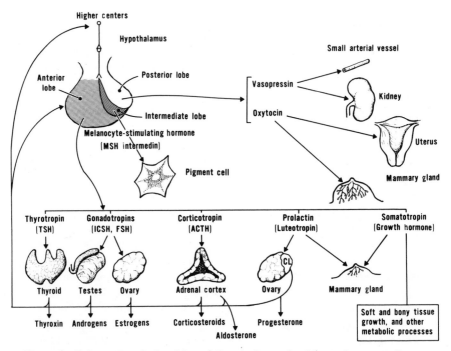

Figure 9: Cybernetic relationships of the pituitary gland (anterior, posterior and intermediate lobes) with the hypothalamus, other endocrine organs, and tissues of the organism. (After Furth; reproduced with the permission of the author.)

proposed by Furth. Theoretically, then, neoplasms of any of the end organs seen in Figure 9 may be produced by some form of manipulation breaking the feedback loop. Conversely, elimination of the end organ may result in specific pituitary neoplasms.

It is also possible to produce neoplasms of the pituitary and the peripheral endocrine organs by the administration of specific hormones. Administration of estrogens in rodents results in pituitary neoplasms that produce prolactin. In the male, Leydig cell neoplasms of the testes can also be induced by the administration of estrogens. While the kidney is not usually considered to be a peripheral endocrine organ, its cells do produce erythropoietin, and estrogen administration can induce renal cortical carcinomas in male hamsters.

In addition to the direct induction of neoplasia by hormonal stimuli, hormones also act in concert with known carcinogenic agents to produce neoplasia. One of the better studied examples of this phenomenon is seen with the induction of mammary adenocarcinomas in rodents. Bittner and others demonstrated three factors essential for the production of mammary carcinoma in mice: genetic susceptibility, hormonal influence, and a virus transmitted through the milk. The first two have been repeatedly demonstrated in a variety of species including humans, but incontrovertible evidence for the participation of a virus in mammary carcinogenesis has been obtained only in mice. In the rat both prolactin and a carcinogen, chemical or physical, have been reported to act together to produce mammary carcinomas. It is also known, however, that chronic treatment with estrogens alone may induce mammary carcinomas in rodents. Thus mammary carcinogenesis in rodents is a very complicated process, possibly requiring several components, these requirements being somewhat variable depending on the species involved.

Hormonal Induction of Cancer in Humans

Until recently the production of neoplasia by endogenous and exogenous hormones had received little attention in the study of human neoplasia, although hormones had been utilized in the therapy of specific types of human cancer, especially that of the breast and prostate. Recently, however, a number of reports, especially those by Herbst and his associates, have demonstrated a relationship between vaginal adenosis and related changes in the vagina of young women exposed to diethylstilbesterol in utero, usually during the first trimester. More ominous is the fact that in a small but significant number of such patients, clear cell adenocarcinoma of the vagina or cervix, and to a lesser extent squamous cell carcinoma of the vagina and cervix, have been demonstrated. Since in at least one study 97% of diethylstilbesterol-exposed young women showed abnormal vaginal findings compared with only 8% in unexposed young women, there is every reason to believe that this estrogenic compound is at least teratogenic if not truly carcinogenic.

That estrogens administered directly to premenopausal women for contraceptive purposes or to postmenopausal women for relief of menopausal symptomatology result in a significant increase in the incidence of liver cancer in the former and endometrial cancer in the latter has now been demonstrated by a number of clinical investigators. In the case of oral contraceptives most of the neoplasms reported are benign hepatic adenomas, but a small yet significant number of carcinomas of the liver have also been found in women receiving this medication for extended periods of time.

Possible Mechanisms
of Hormonal Carcinogenesis

At first glance one might consider that the mechanisms involved in hormonal carcinogenesis are identical with those described for chemical carcinogenesis, i.e., alkylation of nucleic acid, mutation, etc. Endocrine-related neoplasms in humans are not uncommon, as evidenced by carcinoma of the breast and of the prostate. However, there is no evidence to date that hormones, especially steroid hormones, interact directly with nucleic acid, as has been described for the chemical carcinogens. On the other hand, at least one synthetic estrogen has been shown to bind irreversibly to proteins of liver microsomes, probably through an intermediate epoxide form. Thus the possibility has been raised that steroid hormones might interact directly with nucleic acid in the same way chemical carcinogens do. However, polypeptide hormones such as the gonadotropins described earlier exert their action at the cell surface and in all likelihood never reach the nucleus in an undegraded form. Furth suggests that the effect of hormones is merely to increase cell replication and that the rapidly dividing cell thus becomes more susceptible to "endogenous" carcinogenesis from genetic "mistakes" or mutations, the chance of formation of which is increased by the more rapid rate of DNA synthesis. Since this is possible, one should then expect that carcinoma of the small intestine would be a very common neoplasm because of the extremely rapid rate of replication of intestinal epithelial cells. Such is not the case either in humans or in lower forms of life. Unfortunately, then, we are left with a dilemma as to the mechanism of hormonal carcinogenesis. As we shall see later, if one assumes an extragenetic mechanism of the neoplastic transformation akin to an abnormal differentiation, then the mechanisms of hormonal carcinogenesis take on a new appearance.

Radiation Carcinogenesis

Perhaps the first documented example of the induction of neoplasia by high-energy radiation was that of the production of skin cancer by chronic self-exposure to radioactive chemicals by Madame Curie, Roentgen, and their associates. In these cases, the human being was the experimental victim of radiation carcinogenesis. Since radiation is known to have specific mutagenic effects, it has long been assumed that the mechanism of carcinogenesis by high-energy radiation is a partial destruction of or change in the genome. Evidence for this assumption comes from the finding of numerous chromosomal abnormalities in radiation-induced neoplasms. However, Kaplan demonstrated that the radiation induction of leukemia in mice may be completely prevented by the removal of the thymus gland shortly after birth. Furthermore, Kaplan has demonstrated that radiation produces leukemia in these animals by the "activation" of a leukemogenic virus that occurs normally in the specific strain of animals and that is "activated" by the ionizing radiation. More recent data extending those of Kaplan have indicated that the thymus is not only necessary but apparently produces a hormone-like substance that is important in the final genesis of the leukemia. The leukemic cells all originate from the thymus gland.

Studies by Nowell and his collaborators have also demonstrated the interesting phenomenon of the potentiation of carcinogenesis by high-energy radiation when a mitotic stimulus is simultaneously administered to the animal. One of the best examples of this may be seen in the induction of radiation-induced hepatomas in rodents; partial hepatectomy or the administration of sublethal doses of hepatotoxic chemicals such as carbon tetrachloride markedly increases the incidence of hepatomas when radiation is given at specific times in relation to the operation or the administration of the chemical. As we shall see later, this relationship of cell replication to a carcinogenic stimulus is extremely important not only in radiation-induced carcinogenesis but also in chemical and biological carcinogenesis.

There is reasonably good evidence, including the results of chronic exposure to radiation in the early part of this century, that radiation is leukemogenic and carcinogenic in humans. The incidence of leukemia in radiologists in the first half of this century was three to four times that in the general population. Furthermore, continuing studies on the survivors of the atom bomb blasts in Japan show that the incidence of leukemia in persons exposed at the time of the blasts was at least twice as high as that in the general population. Perhaps one of the most unfortunate examples of radiation carcinogenesis in the human being was that found in those workers in the watch industry who utilized pigments containing radium in painting the dials of watches. Many of these individuals absorbed the radioactive ions from the paint, which gave rise to radium deposition in their bones. Within 15 to 25 years after exposure, a number of these individuals appeared with osteogenic sarcomas resulting from the chronic irradiation.

In addition to these, one of the more recently recognized, but in retrospect obvious, examples of radiation-induced cancer is that resulting from the radiation therapy of neoplastic and nonneoplastic disease. [131]I was utilized in the past for the treatment of goiter and other lesions of the thyroid in young individuals. It is now apparent that a significant number of children treated in this way have developed carcinoma of the thyroid in later life.

Thorium dioxide, an alpha emitter, was utilized in a colloidal form to visualize the hepatic parenchyma of the human in vivo. Like the radium dial painters, after a lag of 15 or more years a significant number of patients in which this diagnostic procedure had been utilized developed sarcomas of the liver.

Although it is recognized that radiation itself is carcinogenic, it is used to treat various types of neoplasms. If this type of therapy were not utilized in many patients with cancer, the prognosis for a number of such patients would be quite grave. In the treatment of one relatively benign hematologic cancer, polycythemia vera, early treatment with radioactive phosphate was given in many areas of the world. Recent studies have shown that leukemia resulted in a significant number of patients so treated, especially in those in whom karyotypic abnormalities appeared in bone marrow cells after treatment.

Chronic Irritation Carcinogenesis

Although most textbooks have now dispensed with the general concept that chronic irritation is a carcinogenic stimulus, there still remains the fact that certain conditions in the human being in which chronic inflammation is a constant factor do predispose to neoplasia. Perhaps the best example of this is the chronic draining sinus, usually resulting from osteomyelitis, which, as a result of antibiotics, is relatively rare today. However, in the days when bone infections were rather common, epidermoid carcinomas were found to arise in the skin near chronic draining sinuses. The histology of these regions before the production of the tumor demonstrated a peculiar type of hyperplasia of the squamous epithelium known as pseudoepitheliomatous hyperplasia. Furthermore, it has been suggested that the chronic irritation of the lip produced by smoking a clay pipe can lead to cancer of the lip. However, it is now apparent that many of these examples are considerably more complicated than originally thought, and the concept that chronic irritation per se is sufficient for the carcinogenic stimulus is no longer supported by most oncologists.

References

M. E. Alpert, M. S. R. Hutt, G. N. Wogan, and C. S. Davidson. Association between aflatoxin content of food and hepatoma frequency in Uganda. *Cancer, 28* (1971): 253.

B. N. Ames, W. E. Durston, E. Yamasaki, and F. D. Lee. Carcinogens are mutagens: A simple test system combining liver homogenates for activation and bacteria for detection. *Proc. Natl. Acad. Sci. USA 70* (1973): 2281.

G. T. Beatson. On the treatment of inoperable cases of carcinoma of the mamma: Suggestions for a new method of treatment with illustrative cases. *Lancet 2* (1896): 104.

C. Bernard. *Leçons sur les Phenomenes de la Vie.* J.-B. Baillière et fils, Paris, 2 vol., 1878, 1879.

J. J. Bittner. Mammary cancer in C3H mice of different sublines and their hybrids. *J. Natl. Cancer Inst. 16* (1956): 1263.

H. P. Blejer and W. Wagner. Inorganic arsenic — ambient level approach to the control of occupational cancerigenic exposures. *Ann. N.Y. Acad. Sci. 271* (1976): 179.

K. G. Brand. Induction of sarcomas by subcutaneous implantation of plastics in mice. *Dermat. Dig. 9* (1970): 59.

K. H. Clifton and B. N. Sridharan. Endocrine factors and tumor growth. In *Cancer − A Comprehensive Treatise,* Vol. III (F. F. Becker, ed.). Plenum, New York, 1975, p. 249.

L. J. Cole and P. C. Nowell. Radiation carcinogenesis: The sequence of events. *Science 150* (1965): 1782.

H. A. Edmondson, B. Henderson, and B. Benton. Liver-cell adenomas associated with use of oral contraceptives. *New Eng. J. Med. 294* (1976): 470.

J. Furth. Hormones as etiological agents in neoplasia. In *Cancer – A Comprehensive Treatise,* Vol. I (F. F. Becker, ed.). Plenum, New York, 1975, p. 75.

S. Goldfarb. Sex hormones and hepatic neoplasia. *Cancer Res. 36* (1976): 2584.

C. Heidelberger. Chemical carcinogenesis, chemotherapy: Cancer's continuing core challenge. *Cancer Res. 30* (1970): 1549.

C. Heidelberger. *In vitro* studies on the role of epoxides in carcinogenic hydrocarbon activation. In *Topics in Chemical Carcinogenesis* (W. Nakahara, S. Takayama, T. Sugimura, and S. Odashima, eds.). University of Tokyo Press, 1972, p. 371.

A. L. Herbst, R. J. Kurman, R. E. Scully, and D. C. Poskanzer. Adenocarcinoma of the vagina: Association of maternal stilbestrol therapy with tumor appearance in young women. *New Eng. J. Med. 284* (1971): 878.

K. H. Johnson, L. C. Buoen, I. Brand, and K. G. Brand. Polymer tumorigenesis: Clonal determination of histopathological characteristics during early preneoplasia; relationships to karyotype, mouse strain, and sex. *J. Natl. Cancer Inst. 44* (1970): 785.

H. Kappus and H. Remmer. Metabolic activation of norethisterone (norethindrone) to an irreversibly protein-bound derivative by rate liver microsomes. *Drug. Met. Disp. 3* (1975): 338.

E. C. Kennaway. The identification of a carcinogenic compound in coal-tar. *Brit. Med. J. ii* (1955): 749.

R. Kinosita. Researches on the carcinogenesis of the various chemical substances. *Gann 30* (1936): 423.

F. W. Krüger, G. Walker, and M. Weissler. Carcinogenic action of dimethylnitrosamine in trout not related to methylation of nucleic acids and protein in vivo. *Experientia 26* (1970): 520.

M. W. Lieberman and P. D. Forbes. Demonstration of DNA repair in normal and neoplastic tissues after treatment with proximate chemical carcinogens and ultraviolet radiation. *Nature New Biol. 241* (1973): 199.

M. Lieberman and H. S. Kaplan. Leukemogenic activity of filtrates from radiation-induced lymphoid tumors of mice. *Science 130* (1959): 387.

P. N. Magee and P. F. Swann. Nitroso compounds. *Brit. Med. Bull. 25* (1969): 240.

V. M. Maher, E. C. Miller, J. A. Miller, and W. Szybalski. Mutations and decreases in density of transforming DNA produced by derivatives of the carcinogens 2-acetylaminofluorene and N-methyl-4-aminoazobenzene. *Mol. Pharmacol. 4* (1968): 41.

E. C. Miller and J. A. Miller. Mechanisms of chemical carcinogenesis: Nature of proximate carcinogens and interactions with macromolecules. *Pharmacol. Rev. 18* (1966): 805.

J. A. Miller. Carcinogenesis by chemicals: An overview. *Cancer Res. 30* (1970): 559.

R. W. Miller. Radiation-induced cancer. *J. Natl. Cancer Inst. 49* (1972): 1221.

R. W. Miller. Transplacental chemical carcinogenesis in man. *J. Natl. Cancer Inst. 47* (1971): 1169.

R. A. Peters. Mechanism of the toxicity of the active constituent of *Dichapetalum cymosum* and related compounds. *Adv. Enzymol. 18* (1957): 113.

H. J-P. Ryser. Chemical carcinogenesis. *New Eng. J. Med. 285* (1971): 721.

T. Sasaki and T. Yoshida. Experimentelle Erzeugung des Lebercarcinoms durch Fütterung mit o-Amidoazotoluol. *Virchow's Arch. Path. Anat. 295* (1935): 175.

A. M. Schmidt, W. V. Whitehorn, and E. W. Martin. Estrogens and endometrial cancer. *FDA Drug Bull. 6* (1976): 18.

S. Sorof, E. M. Young, and M. G. Ott. Soluble liver h proteins during hepatocarcinogenesis by aminoazo dyes and 2-acetylaminofluorene in the rat. *Cancer Res. 18* (1958): 33.

A. Stafl, and R. F. Mattingly. Vaginal adenosis: A precancerous lesion. *Am. J. Ob. and Gynecol. 120* (1975): 666.

N. E. Stinson. The tissue reaction induced in rats and guinea pigs by polymethlymethacrylate (acrylic) and stainless steel. *Brit. J. Exp. Pathol. 45* (1964): 21.

T. Sugimoto and H. Terayama. Studies on carcinogen-binding proteins. I. Isolation and characterization of aminoazo dye-bound protein after administration of a single large dose of 3'-methyl-4-dimethylaminoazobenzene to rats. *Biochim. Biophys. Acta 214* (1970): 533.

J. H. Weisburger and G. M. Williams. Metabolism of chemical carcinogens. In *Cancer*, Vol. 1 (F. F. Becker, ed.). Plenum, New York, 1975, p. 185.

K. Yamagiwa and K. Ichikawa. Experimentelle Studie über die Pathogenese der Epithelialgeschwülste. *Mitteilungen Med. Facultät Kaiserl. Univ. Tokyo 15* (1915): 295.

4

The Etiology of Cancer: Biological Factors

Infectious Agents as Causes of Cancer

In 1907 Fibiger reported the occurrence of papillomas of the stomach in rats infected with a small parasitic worm. Fibiger showed that the cockroach was the intermediate host of this worm and that by feeding normal rats a diet infected with cockroaches, he could apparently produce papillomas of the stomach. In the 1920s Fibiger was awarded the Nobel Prize for this work. Unfortunately, one year thereafter his experiments were shown to be invalid. Partly as a result of these studies and the publicity attached to them, biological factors in cancer causation became an unpopular topic for the experimental oncologist.

Despite this setback, over the years numerous investigators have reported that certain biological factors are important in the causation of cancer. The parasitic worm, *Spirocerca lupi,* is associated with esophageal sarcomas in the dog. Studies have demonstrated that the worms encyst in the wall of the esophagus, and around this cyst a sarcoma may arise. In addition, the parasite, cysticercus, has been shown to produce hepatic sarcomas in the rat. A possibly comparable disease in the human is seen as a result of infestation by the parasitic worm, schistosoma. In addition to multicellular parasites, in some forms of life unicellular organisms have been associated with neoplasia. The best example of this is the production of crown gall tumors in plants by infection with the bacterium, *Agrobacter tumifaciens.* The exact mechanism whereby the bacterium induces this neoplasm is not certain, but recent evidence has suggested that a large plasmid in the bacterium is essential for tumor-inducing ability and part of it is actually transferred to the plant cell during its neoplastic conversion.

46

Intracellular parasites have long been implicated as the cause of certain types of neoplasms. In 1904 Ellerman and Bang demonstrated a viral causation for avian leukosis. In 1911 Rous reported that cell-free extracts of sarcomas in chickens would in some instances produce sarcomas when injected into other chickens. In 1928 Shope described the Shope papilloma virus of rabbits, and in the latter 1930s the Bittner mammary tumor virus was discovered. However, the general significance and importance of viruses in the causation of cancer was not appreciated until after the discovery of lysogeny in bacteria and the importance of latency in viral infections. In the early 1950s Gross reported that injection of cell-free filtrates from AKR mice with leukemia into newborn AKR mice would result in a high percentage of leukemia at a later period in the life of the inoculated animals. Since Gross's experiments, numerous individuals have extended these studies, and considerable biological knowledge is now available on the viral causation of tumors.

Oncogenic DNA Viruses

Oncogenic viruses may be divided into two general classes, the DNA viruses and the RNA viruses. Oncogenic DNA viruses include the papovaviruses, to which the polyoma virus of the mouse and the simian virus 40 (SV40) belong; the adenoviruses, several of which are causative agents of upper respiratory infections in the human; and the herpesviruses. The latter class of viruses is much larger, with a much more complex genome than that found in the papova or the adeno virus families. Some characteristics and the relative size of the known classes of oncogenic viruses are seen in Figure 10. In general, infection of cells with oncogenic DNA viruses can lead to two possible alternatives: the cells may die with the release of newly formed virus, or the cells may become transformed into neoplastic cells, with little or no virus production resulting from these transformed cells (see Figure 11). The molecular weights of the viral DNAs of these three classes of viruses are 3×10^6 for the papova group, $20\text{-}25 \times 10^6$ for the adeno group, and 1×10^8 for the herpesviruses. The DNA of the papovavirus is circular, whereas that of the other groups is linear. During infection of cells by DNA tumor viruses, the papovavirus DNA integrates into the genome of the parasitized cell. This integration occurs in the transformed cells and also during a lytic replicative cycle of the virus. In the transformed cell several copies of papovavirus DNA may be found associated with the cellular genome, although the exact number of gene equivalents per cell varies among different cell populations. In the case of adenoviruses, there is evidence of integration of viral DNA into cellular

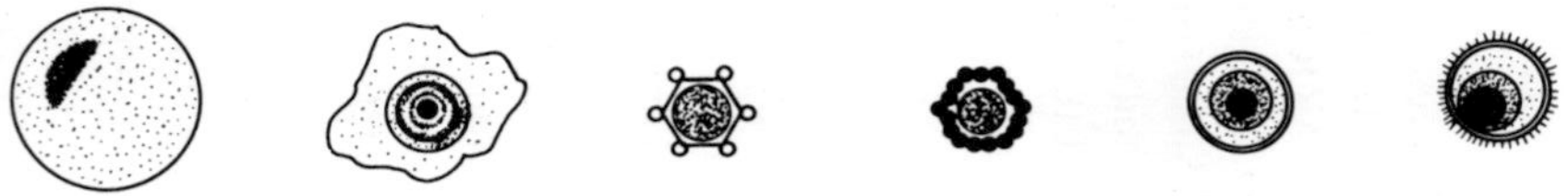

	Papilloma-Myxoma viruses	Herpes-viruses (EBV, Lucké HSV-2)	Adenoviruses	Papovaviruses (SV-40, Poly-oma, JC, BK)	Rous sarcoma virus (C-type particle)	Mammary tumor virus (B-type particle)
M.W. of GENOME	$160 \times 10^6 (?)$	100×10^6	$20\text{--}25 \times 10^6$	3×10^6	$3 \times 2 \times 10^6$	$3 \times 2 \times 10^6 (?)$
CODING POTENTIAL (Calculated number of polypeptides)	—	100	23	3	?(?)	?(?)

Figure 10: Artist's conception of the relative size and ultrastructural appearance in thin sections of viruses known to be oncogenic in birds and mammals. The question marks indicate that the value presented is not absolutely firm.

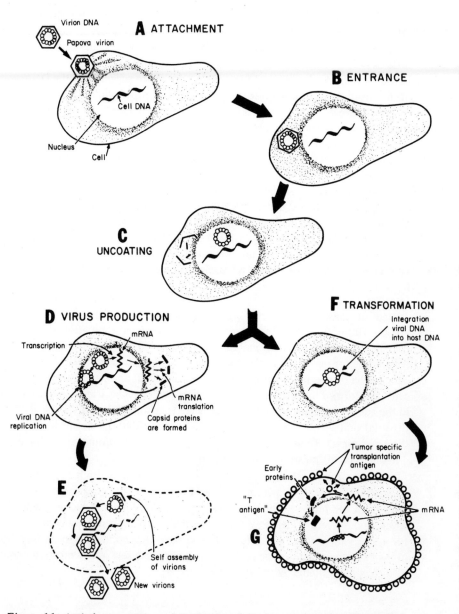

Figure 11: Artist's conception of the interaction of an oncogenic papovavirus with a susceptible cell. The two pathways of lysis and transformation are denoted separately. (After Allen and Cole, reproduced with permission.)

DNA during the replicative cycle of the virus. In the adenovirus-transformed cell at least some bits of the viral genome are stably maintained. It is of interest, however, that evidence has been presented that only a small segment, as little as 4-5%, of the total adenovirus genome may induce transformation in rodent cells. At the moment there is no evidence to suggest that the DNA of the entire genome of herpesviruses integrates into the cellular DNA during the replicative cycle. However, cells transformed by herpesviruses do contain viral genomes, in some instances more than 50 such copies within the nucleus of the transformed cell. At present, however, it does not appear that this association is by integration, although a small amount of integrated virus has been reported.

Although virus replication does not occur to any significant degree in cells transformed by oncogenic DNA viruses, substantial evidence has been obtained by means of nucleic acid hybridization that integrated viral information is transcribed within the transformed cell. Most of this transcription is of the "early" viral genes, whose products are not the capsid proteins of the virus and about which we know relatively little. However, one of the products resulting from the early transcription of papovavirus-transformed cells is the so-called T antigen. This appears to consist of two proteins that occur in the nucleus of transformed cells, having a molecular weight in the native state of 90,000. During lytic growth this protein(s) is involved in the initiation of each round of viral DNA synthesis and, in the transformed cell, the T antigen is responsible for maintaining the transformed state. A similar antigen also occurs in adenovirus-transformed cells, and an analogous antigen may be seen in cells transformed by herpesviruses. It is of interest that the T antigen occurs in the adenovirus-transformed cells that were transformed by only 1-6% of the total viral genome. Furthermore, in the case of SV40-transformed cells, the genes for the T antigen appear to be associated with chromosome number 7 in one class of transformed human cells.

In addition to the T antigen, a surface or S antigen is also induced by oncogenic DNA virus transformation (see Figure 11). This S antigen is distinct from the tumor-specific transplantation antigen about which we will speak later. Recent evidence also indicates that the S antigen is not coded for by the viral genome, but is related to antigens that normally appear only in the embryonic state of the cell; this indicates some sort of derepression of the cellular genome by the viral infection.

Oncogenic RNA Viruses

Strongly transforming RNA viruses act somewhat differently from the DNA tumor viruses in that upon infection the cell is not killed, but is usually transformed. In most instances the transformed cell then continues to produce more of the virus (Figure 12). The most famous example of an oncogenic RNA virus is the Rous sarcoma virus, which produces mesenchymal neoplasms in birds. Recently this virus has been shown to infect several mammalian species as well. The Rous sarcoma virus is a member of a group of viruses termed *retroviruses.* Temin's classification of the retroviruses is seen in Table 3. These viruses have within their virion an RNA-directed DNA polymerase, which has been termed "reverse transcriptase." This enzyme was discovered simultaneously by Drs. H. M. Temin and S. Mizutani in the McArdle Laboratory and by Dr. D. Baltimore of M.I.T. Many viruses possessing the gene for "reverse transcriptase" are oncogenic, but some are not. In addition, numerous C-type retroviruses have been described for which no known pathogenicity has been demonstrated.

For convenience it is possible to divide the oncogenic retroviruses into three general classes: sarcoma viruses, leukemia viruses, and mammary tumor viruses. Morphologically the virions are enclosed in an envelope derived from the modified plasma membrane of the host cell (see Figure 12). The nucleic acid is present in a nucleoid, which contains not only the viral genome but also some low molecular weight RNAs separate from the genome. The nucleoid contains a 70S RNA, which is the viral genome and which is diploid, consisting of two roughly equal components, each of a molecular weight of approximately 3 million. The sarcoma and leukosis viruses are of the C-type, whereas the mammary tumor viruses are of the B-type. These are morphologic terms, distinguished by the eccentricity of the nucleoid and prominent protruding spikes on the virion envelope of the B-type particle, with the C-type exhibiting a centrally placed nucleoid and less prominent spikes (Figure 10).

The replication of oncogenic RNA viruses differs somewhat from that of the DNA oncogenic viruses, basically because of the nature of the genome of the virus. In the case of retroviruses, transformation requires the formation of a DNA copy of the viral genome, which is then integrated into the genome of the host cell. Subsequently, transcription of the

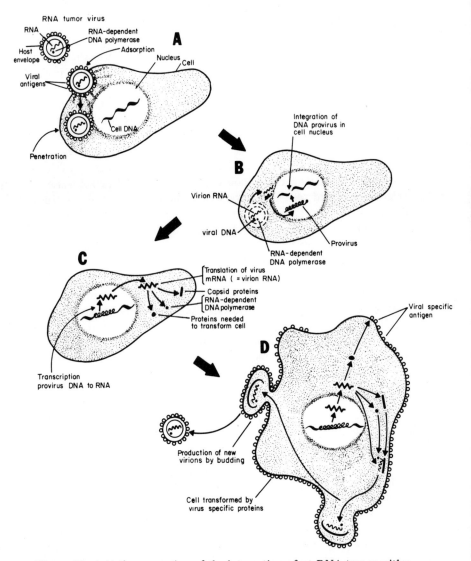

Figure 12: Artist's conception of the interaction of an RNA tumor with a susceptible cell. The production of new virions by budding of the cell surface and the absence of cell killing by the virus is denoted. (After Allen and Cole, reproduced with permission of the authors.)

Table 3.[a] Classification of Retroviruses

1. Avian leukosis-sarcoma viruses

2. Reticuloendotheliosis viruses

3. Mammalian C-type retroviruses
   a. Mouse C-type retroviruses
   b. Feline C-type retroviruses
   c. Rat C-type retroviruses
   d. Hamster C-type retroviruses
   e. Simian C-type retroviruses
   f. RD-114-like C-type retroviruses
   g. Murine, feline, simian sarcoma viruses

4. Viper C-type retroviruses

5. Mouse mammary tumor viruses

6. Mason-Pfizer monkey viruses

7. Visna viruses

8. Syncytium-forming viruses

9. Particles related to retroviruses.

[a]After Temin (1974).

integrated viral genome leads to the constant production of virus by the transformed cell. In some cases the viral genome is defective and transcription of the integrated viral genome does not give all viral products and thus no production of virus, although the cell is transformed. Virus production may be reinstated by infection with another "helper" virus, which usually belongs to the same general group of viruses. In some instances it is only through relatively heroic means, such as somatic cell hybridization or treatment with BUdR, that virus production by the cell can occur.

Viral or virus-induced antigens (proteins) of cells transformed by RNA tumor viruses are somewhat more complex than those transformed by DNA tumor viruses. Group-specific antigens are those shared by all related retroviruses derived from a single host species, with determinants located on at least two polypeptides in the core of the virion. In addition, there are type-specific antigens, which appear to be located on the glycoproteins of the spikes on the virion. The transformed cells exhibit a tumor-specific transplantation antigen, about which we will learn more later.

The mammary tumor virus is somewhat unique in that its oncogenicity is absolutely dependent on the host hormonal environment, primarily because the development of the mammary gland is dependent on hormones. Thus the virus, although present in cells in the male, seldom expresses its oncogenicity in that sex principally because of the hormonal environment, which does not allow differentiation of the mammary gland as seen in the female. On the other hand, in the mouse there is reasonable evidence that most strains in the laboratory are infected by this virus and that it may be activated in females by aging, irradiation, or other chemicals including hormones. Earlier studies indicated that the virus is passed in the milk from mother to offspring.

Endogenous Viruses and
the Neoplastic Transformation

One of the most controversial subjects in viral oncology is the question of whether or not chemical carcinogens may activate a latent oncogenic virus, this being the primary mechanism through which the chemicals act rather than their exerting a direct effect on macromolecular syntheses or interactions within the cell. A theory proposed by Huebner, which has been termed the "oncogene" theory, states that the information for oncogenic RNA viruses is inherent in the genome and is transmitted vertically. Recently Temin has pointed out that this is not true in the case of avian leukosis and sarcoma viruses and may well not be true for most mammalian cells. On the other hand, evidence for endogenous virus genes of weakly oncogenic viruses has been forthcoming from inbred mice in several laboratories, and recently Rowe has presented evidence of viral-genetic information in the chromosomes of very early embryonic cells of the AKR strain of mice. Furthermore, the appearance of C-type particles in cells and the general ubiquitous nature of this type of virus add some support for this general concept. In fact, recent studies by Huebner and his associates have demonstrated evidence for C-type virus particles in neoplasms produced in several rodent species by chemical carcinogens. Still the oncogene hypothesis is by no means proved and may have only limited application.

Hereditary Factors in the Etiology of Cancer

Many individuals have suggested that cancer is a hereditary disease. It is safe to say today that with relatively few exceptions, some of which are touched on later, cancer is not a hereditary disease but is acquired. However, this is not to say that neoplasia may not have as its common denominator changes in the genome. Furthermore, the evidence that many types of cancer have some degree of genetic predisposition in combination with a variety of environmental factors is now well known. Therefore, although few neoplasms exhibit a clearly defined pattern of heredity, polygenic or multifactorial inheritance undoubtedly plays a significant role in increasing the risk of cancer for a large number of human beings.

Dominant and Recessive Disorders
Associated with High Incidences of Cancer

While the number of cases of cancer having a definite genetic mode of inheritance is small relative to the incidence of the disease in general, a variety of autosomal disorders, both dominant and recessive, that are associated with or clearly causative of specific neoplasms is seen in Table 4.

In viewing the variety of diseases seen in Table 4, one will notice that virtually all of the autosomal dominant disorders have as a major part of their clinical findings the appearance of a specific type of neoplasm. Familial multiple polyposis of the colon is an autosomal dominant disease of the human. The lesion consists of myriads of polyps over the entire mucosa of the colon, sometimes extending into upper levels of the intestinal tract. Polyps appear before the second and third decades of life, and it has been clearly shown that, if the lesion is of long duration, malignant neoplasms will develop from the benign polyps. A related disease is the Peutz-Jeghers syndrome, which is characterized by polyps of the entire gastrointestinal tract as well as melanin pigmentation of the buccal mucosa and fingers. Another neoplasm that arises in infants and children, the retinoblastoma, when bilateral, is inherited as a Mendelian dominant. The "cancer family syndrome" that was described in the early part of this century is associated predominantly with cancer of the colon and uterus. This syndrome is different from the isolated cancer "families" and sporadic foci of patients with neoplasia that have been suggested as evidence for the infectious nature of

---

Table 4. Cancer and Precancerous Diseases with a Distinct Hereditary Pattern

1. *Autosomal-dominant disorders*
   Familial polyposis coli
   Multiple cutaneous cysts, osteomas, and polyposis coli
     (Gardner's syndrome)
   Hereditary exostosis
   Nevoid basal cell carcinoma syndrome
   Phaeochromocytoma
   Hereditary polyendocrine adenomatosis
   Medullary thyroid carcinoma, bilateral, with amyloid production
     and pheochromocytoma
   Intraocular melanoma
   Familial gastrointestinal polyposis and mucocutaneous pigmentation
     (Peutz-Jeghers syndrome)
   Tylosis (keratosis palmaris et plantaris) and esophageal cancer
   Neurofibromatosis (von Recklinghausen's disease)
   Retinoblastoma
   Carotid body tumors
   Cerebelloretinal hemangioblastomatosis (Lindau-von Hippel disease)
   Tuberous sclerosis
   Cancer families

2. *Autosomal-recessive disorders*
   Xeroderma pigmentosum
   Bloom's syndrome
   Fanconi's aplastic anemia
   Decreased pigmentation, photophobia, nystagmus, and leukocytic
     inclusions (Chediak-Higashi syndrome)
   Dermatitis and thrombocytopenic purpura (Wiskott-Aldrich syndrome)
   Ataxia-telangiectasis (Louis-Barr syndrome)

---

certain types of neoplasms. While other types of neoplasms occur in the cancer family syndrome, the incidence of endometrial and colonic cancer predominates as do multiple primary malignancies occurring at an early age.

On the other hand, autosomal recessive disorders associated with neoplasia, which are listed in Table 4 as well, are mostly, though not entirely, associated with special defects in DNA metabolism or chromosomal structure.

The lack of ability of cells from patients with xeroderma pigmentosum to repair ultraviolet damage to their DNA is now well known. In addition, recent studies have indicated that related genetic lesions occur in Bloom's syndrome, Fanconi's anemia, and the Louis-Barr syndrome.

In general, the autosomal-dominant disorders associated with neoplasia are virtually all characterized by multiple primary neoplasms. This is not to say that every patient with multiple primaries exhibits hereditary neoplasia. However, in those neoplasms of duplicate organs, i.e., adrenals, kidney, breast, eye, etc. as well as organs exhibiting both right and left sections, bilateral neoplasia is usually a sign of an autosomal-dominant disorder.

A Genetic Model for Inherited
and Spontaneous Cancer

Although the available evidence indicates that the diseases listed in Table 4 exhibit the pattern of inheritance shown, because of the rarity of most of these conditions it is at times difficult to be absolutely certain. However, the hereditary pattern of most of these conditions has been rather solidly established. Recently Knudson has suggested an interesting model to relate the hereditary and nonhereditary forms of a specific neoplasm.

Knudson's model suggests that, in order for a neoplasm of one of these types to be produced, two genetic mutations must occur. If the first mutation is prezygotic, i.e., present in the germ cell prior to fertilization, the neoplasm is then scored as hereditary. When the first mutation is postzygotic, the neoplasm is nonhereditary and usually occurs only as a single neoplasm in the patient. This is due to the fact that the probability is extremely small that an individual would acquire both mutations in more than one cell in the body. Therefore, by this thesis virtually all bilateral or multiple primary neoplasms of the same tissue are hereditary, whereas unilateral or single neoplasms of a tissue are mostly nonhereditary with an occasional hereditary case. This theory works quite well for certain types of hereditary neoplasms in humans, such as the retinoblastoma, but is not consistent with all of the data available in other neoplasms such as Wilms' tumor and, of course, many of the "nonhereditary" types of neoplasms. Still, the model does account for the high incidence of bilateral neoplasms in children, since one would expect that the second mutational event, if it occurs at random, would occur more frequently than the two mutations needed for a spontaneous neoplasm.

Genetics and Environment
in the Causation of Cancer

While the list of genetic neoplasms and genetic diseases associated with a high incidence of neoplasia (Table 4) represents only a tiny fraction of the total incidence of neoplasia, there is evidence that some of the more common types of neoplasms in humans do exhibit a genetic predisposition and, in a few instances, specific genetic inheritance. The best example of this is seen in cancer of the breast in women. Extensive studies on mammary cancer in rodents have suggested a variety of potential environmental interactions with the genetic apparatus that can ultimately lead to the neoplastic transformation. Although there is no substantial evidence as yet for a specific mammary tumor virus in humans, nor is there evidence for any transmission of such a putative virus through the milk, there are certain conditions in the mouse that offer potential models for the transmission of mammary cancer in humans. One RNA virus in mice, the nodule-inducing virus (NIV), is transmitted through the male as readily as through the female but not through the milk, while another is transmitted by both sexes as well as through the milk. Such models clearly have their potential counterparts in human breast cancer. Furthermore, since there is considerable evidence that the mammary tumor virus in mice is transmitted as a provirus, i.e., vertically through the genome of the mouse, it may be transmitted as a dominant gene. There is now considerable evidence in humans that bilateral mammary cancer in women prior to age 40 has all the characteristics of an autosomal-dominant pattern of inheritance.

If one separates breast cancer patients into premenopausal and post-menopausal cases, then one finds that the incidence of breast cancer in relatives of the premenopausal group is threefold higher than that of the average population, but there is no increased incidence in the relatives of the post-menopausal group. This may be related to the inheritance pattern of the bilateral breast cancer patient prior to age 40. Furthermore, one may also expect that such young breast cancer patients might have the greatest chance of demonstrating any putative breast cancer virus in humans.

Since the majority of colon cancer in this country does not appear to be directly genetic in origin, numerous studies have been directed toward showing genetic factors in the relatively common adenocarcinoma of the colon not associated with polyposis. The evidence to date does not show any simple genetic pattern of inheritance but indicates that if a predisposition occurs it is probably polygenic. On the other hand, while there is no evidence for a specific gene relationship with leukemia, there is good evidence to suggest that a number of cases of leukemia may have exhibited a significant predisposition to the disease. The groups that are at greatest risk are listed in Table 5. One of the most interesting aspects of this table is that when one of identical twins has leukemia, although the risk is about 20% that the unaffected twin will succumb to the disease, 80% of such individuals do not appear to be at risk.

There are many obvious animal models of leukemia, especially those associated with oncogenic viruses. One of the best examples of genetic factors in neoplastic development is seen in the genesis of leukemia in inbred strains of mice. The susceptibility of these animals to the Friend virus, a typical oncogenic RNA virus, has been shown to be the result of a multiple-gene trait. In particular, a locus in the host's genome termed the FV-1 locus significantly affects the susceptibility of the host to the virus. Furthermore, other studies have demonstrated that at least two alleles of this locus occur. On the basis of these findings one may separate mouse strains into two types depending on which of the two alleles is present in their genome. These two types of animals are called the N-type and the B-type. It is possible to characterize viruses by whether they are N-tropic or B-tropic, i.e., whether the virus

Table 5. Groups at Exceptionally High Risk of Leukemia[a]

Group	Approximate Risk	Time Interval to Onset
Identical twin of children with leukemia	1 in 5[b]	Weeks or months
Radiation-treated polycythemia vera	1 in 6	10-15 years
Bloom's syndrome	1 in 8[c]	30 years of age
Hiroshima survivors who were within 1,000 meters of the hypocenter	1 in 60	12 years
Down's syndrome	1 in 95	10 years of age
Radiation-treated patients with ankylosing spondylitis	1 in 270	15 years
Sibs of leukemic children	1 in 720	10 years
U.S. Caucasian children 15 years of age	1 in 2,880	10 years

[a]After Miller.

[b]Of 22 sets of identical twins with leukemia, the co-twin was affected in five instances.

[c]Three leukemics among 23 persons with Bloom's syndrome.

replicates in NIH (N-type) mice or in BALB/c (B-type) mice, respectively. Thus the gene is quite important for the susceptibility of specific mouse strains to certain RNA oncogenic viruses. Furthermore, this gene and others are important in the expression of endogenous viruses, i.e., those transmitted through the genome, such as are seen in the AKR mouse strain. As yet, however, no specific genetic loci have been demonstrated to be associated with the appearance of or resistance to the presence of leukemia in humans.

Somatic Mutations as a Factor in Neoplasia

In view of the fact that most neoplasms are not related to a specific genetic alteration, although there is ample circumstantial evidence for a mutational event as the principal factor in the genesis of neoplasia, a variety of studies have been directed toward the possibility that neoplasia results from a direct genetic mutation in the adult. This mutation has been termed a *somatic mutation,* which is taken to mean any hereditary trait occurring in cells of the mature organism. This definition does not require that the heritably transmitted change necessarily be due to an alteration in the genome itself, but it may be the result of epigenetic alterations as well.

At our present state of knowledge it is probably more plausible that any existent genetic mechanism for the neoplastic transformation of the vast majority of neoplasms in the adult exhibits a polygenic mode of inheritance. Such a mechanism would of course include as a possible corollary excess genetic information such as may be seen in many aneuploid neoplasms. The diversity of karyotypes seen even in a single neoplasm, especially as a neoplasm progresses from a high degree of differentiation to a poorly differentiated tumor, might account for the heterogeneity characteristic of neoplasia in general and any·one neoplasm specifically. On the other hand, some studies that have been carried out in neoplasms that progressed from euploid to aneuploid states do not show any significant phenotypic changes. In the last analysis, however, numerous studies have also demonstrated that, while primary neoplasms may be euploid, tumor progression is almost always accompanied by karyotypic changes in the total population leading to aneuploidy (Chapter 6).

A major line of evidence for the occurrence of somatic mutations in neoplasia is the appearance of chromosomal abnormalities in tumors. Although certain benign as well as malignant neoplasms possess morphologically normal karyotypes, aneuploidy (an abnormal karyotype not possessing a whole number multiple of the normal haploid chromosomal content) is the rule rather than the exception. The major dilemma, however, is whether or not the changes in karyotype are the result or the cause of the neoplasia.

Quantitatively, neoplasia is a disease of the aged, and there is ample evidence to indicate that aneuploidy increases in cellular populations in vivo with the age of the individual. Furthermore, chronic radiation, which predisposes to neoplasms, also increases the frequency of chromosomal abnormalities. In one specific neoplasm, chronic myeloid leukemia, a specific chromosomal change has been quite definitely associated with the tumor. This neoplasm is of leukocytes and, in a significant percentage of the cases (about 25%), is associated with an abnormality in chromosome number 22. The abnormality appears to be a shortening of the long arm of the chromosome. This has been termed the "Philadelphia" chromosome, after the city where it was first described. It has been reported to occur in a number of individuals who do not have chronic myeloid leukemia, but almost invariably these individuals at a later time exhibit the disease. In this instance there is reasonably good evidence that the chromosomal change preceded the actual neoplasm. Recent evidence through the use of banding techniques has indicated that the Philadelphia chromosome is actually the result of a translocation of the distal portion of the long arm of chromosome 22 to the end of the long arm of chromosome 9 or rarely to other chromosomes rather than a deletion. It is of interest in this connection that there is a higher incidence of leukemia in the trisomy, i.e., three copies of a chromosome rather than the two normally present in the diploid cell. In addition to Down's syndrome, several other diseases are known to be associated with chromosomal "instability." Two such diseases, Bloom's and Fanconi's syndromes, are associated with an extremely high incidence of cancer in affected individuals.

Recent advances in the technology of karyotyping (which involves the differential staining of individual chromosomes) have opened an entirely new vista in the relationship of somatic mutations to the neoplastic transformation. Some neoplasms, whose karyotypes were shown to be very similar to or essentially identical with the normal karyotype by the old methodologies, have now been shown to exhibit abnormalities including translocations and deletions of segments of chromosomes. However, in some series of experimental tumors, such as the hepatocellular carcinomas, perfectly normal karyotypes have been described, even when studied by the new banding techniques.

A number of other neoplastic conditions have also been associated with rather specific chromosome abnormalities. Some of these are listed in Table 6. In this table can be seen several conditions associated with chromosomal abnormalities, including the association of chronic myelogenous

Table 6. Identification of Specific Chromosome Abnormalities in Various Neoplastic Diseases

Disease	Number of patients examined	Total with specific abnormality	Abnormality observed[a]
CML			
Chronic phase	23	23	9q+,22a−(Ph[1])
Acute phase	5	5	+8
	8	8	+ marker 17q
	5	4	Two Ph[1]
Acute myeloblastic leukemia in females	3	2	45, X, t(8;21)(q22;q22)
Polycythemia vera	6	6	20q−
Myelodysplasia	2	2	+8
Meningioma	10	8+	−22
	5	3	−8
Burkitt's lymphoma	12	10	14q+

[a]+, additional; −, absent; q, long arm; t, translocation. (See Rowley, 1974, for further definitions of chromosome abnormalities.)

leukemia with the Philadelphia chromosome. Among the most consistent and better known examples shown is the deletion of chromosome 22 in meningiomas. In addition, an extra band has been found at the end of the long arm of chromosome 14 in cells and cell lines from Burkitt's lymphomas. The remaining diseases listed in Table 6 have a somewhat variable chromosome pattern, although the patients listed did exhibit the changes noted. Therefore, a consistent chromosome pattern is seen only with most cases of chronic myelogenous leukemia, meningioma, and Burkitt's lymphoma. In the case of these three, one may therefore suggest that the somatic mutation resulting in the chromosomal abnormality preceded or coincided with the actual appearance of the disease in the patient. All other chromosomal patterns with neoplastic disease have shown significant variability, although in any specific neoplasm, exemplified especially by the leukemias, one may be able to recognize a "stem line" with a specific karyotype which predominates in that particular neoplasm.

While this extreme variation in karyotype of neoplasms, with the exception of the three mentioned above, is characteristic of the disease, an interesting finding has recently been reported in a number of established neoplastic cell lines maintained in vitro. Each of these cell lines has a relatively diverse number of karyotypes, yet the DNA content of each cell is relatively constant and varies little from a mode for the whole culture. This suggests that in the far-advanced neoplastic cell the chromosomes and their components may be interchanged during interphase, resulting in a variety of morphologic karyotypes evident at mitosis. Such a flexible interchange of chromosomal components is not found in normal or aging cells. What the significance of this phenomenon is to our understanding of the nature of the neoplastic state is not apparent at this time.

Neoplasia as a Disease of Cell Differentiation

Although the broad definition of somatic mutation perhaps encompasses cell differentiation, relatively few oncologists have considered neoplasia as an abnormal differentiation. It is likely that the process of cell differentiation in the development of multicellular organisms does not involve a series of directed genetic mutations. Rather, the heritable phenotypes that occur during differentiation are associated with alterations in the regulation of genetic expression of a genome identical in all cells of the organism. The mechanisms of cell differentiation are obscure, and thus the study of neoplasia as an abnormality in this process has of necessity been rather slow.

Recently, however, through the studies of Mintz and also of Gardner and his associates, the potential importance of considering neoplasia as a disease of differentiation has taken on new significance. In the experiments of these investigators blastulas (Figure 6) inoculated with malignant teratoma cells were shown to develop into normal mice without any neoplastic cells but exhibited cellular populations from both the normal parents and the neoplastic teratoma cells, which had originated from a genetically distinct mouse line. These experiments clearly demonstrate that under the appropriate environmental conditions neoplastic cells can be made to revert back to a normal phenotype and to lose all characteristics of the neoplastic transformation. The interested reader is referred to the papers by Mintz, Gardner, and others for further details of these experiments. Such experiments demonstrate that at least in the mouse teratoma and possibly in a number of other neoplasms as well, the neoplastic phenotype may be a result of an abnormal differentiation and expression of a normal genome rather than the expression and differentiation of an abnormal genome.

References

D. W. Allen, and P. Cole. Viruses and human cancer. *New Eng. J. Med. 286* (1972): 70, 82.

D. Baltimore. RNA-dependent DNA polymerase in virions of RNA tumor viruses. *Nature 226* (1970): 1209.

F. F. Becker (ed.). *Cancer – A Comprehensive Treatise, Vol. 2: Viral Carcinogenesis.* Plenum, New York, 1975.

T. Boveri. *Zur Frage der Entstehung maligner Tumoren,* Gustav Fisher, Jena, 1914.

Chromosome structure and function. *Cold Spring Harbor Symp. Quant. Biol. 38,* 1974.

C. M. Croce, and H. Koprowski. Assignment of gene(s) for cell transformation to human chromosome 7 carrying the simian virus 40 genome. *Proc. Natl. Acad. Sci. USA 72* (1975): 1658.

A. E. Freeman, G. J. Kelloff, M. L. Vernon, W. T. Lane, W. I. Capps, S. D. Bumgarner, H. C. Turner, and R. J. Huebner. Prevalence of endogenous type-C virus in normal hamster tissues and hamster tumors induced by chemical carcinogens, simian virus 40, and polyoma virus. *J. Natl. Cancer Inst. 52* (1974): 1469.

R. C. Gallo. RNA-dependent DNA polymerase in viruses and cells: Views on the current state. *Blood 39* (1972): 117.

J. German (ed.). *Chromosomes and Cancer.* Wiley, New York, 1974.

J. German. Genes which increase chromosomal instability in somatic cells and predispose to cancer. *Prog. Med. Genet. 8* (1972): 61.

F. L. Graham, A. J. van der Eb, and H. L. Heijneker. Size and location of the transforming region in human adenovirus type 5 DNA. *Nature 251* (1974): 687.

I. Granberg. Chromosomes in preinvasive, microinvasive and invasive cervical carcinoma. *Heredita 68* (1971): 165.

R. Hand and J. German. A retarded rate of DNA chain growth in Bloom's syndrome. *Proc. Natl. Acad. Sci. USA 72* (1975): 758.

W. E. Heston. The genetic aspects of human cancer. *Adv. Cancer Res. 23* (1976): 1.

W. E. Heston and G. Vlahakis. Factors in the causation of spontaneous hepatomas in mice. *J. Natl. Cancer Inst. 37* (1966): 839.

C. S. Hill, M. L. Ibanez, N. A. Samaan, M. J. Aheran, and R. L. Clark. Medullary (solid) carcinoma of the thyroid gland: An analysis of the M. D. Anderson Hospital experience with patients with the tumor, its special features and its histogenesis. *Medicine 52* (1973): 141.

M. Hill and J. Hillova. RNA and DNA forms of the genetic material of C-type viruses and the integrated state of the DNA form in the cellular chromosome. *Biochim. Biophys. Acta 355* (1974): 7.

R. J. Huebner and G. J. Todaro. Oncogenes of RNA tumor viruses as determinants of cancer. *Proc. Natl. Acad. Sci. USA 64* (1969): 1087.

J. H. Joncas. Clinical significance of the EB herpes virus infection in man. *Progr. Med. Virol. 14* (1972): 200.

P. M. Karemer, L. L. Deaven, H. A. Crissman, J. A. Steinkamp, and D. F. Petersen. On the nature of heteroploidy. *Cold Spring Harbor Symp. Quant. Biol. 38* (1974): 133.

H. Kato. Induction of sister chromatid exchanges by chemical mutagens and its possible relevance to DNA repair. *Exp. Cell Res. 85* (1974): 239.

G. Klein. Herpes viruses and oncogenesis. *Proc. Natl. Acad. Sci. USA 69* (1972): 1056.

A. G. Knudson. Genetics and the etiology of childhood cancer. *Pediat. Res. 10* (1976): 513.

A. G. Knudson and L. C. Strong. Mutation and cancer: Neuroblastoma and phenochromocytoma. *Ann. J. Human Gen. 24* (1972): 514.

A. G. Knudson, H. W. Hethcote, and B. W. Brown. Mutation and childhood cancer: A probabilistic model for the incidence of retinoblastoma. *Proc. Natl. Acad. Sci. USA 72* (1975): 5116.

F. Lilly. Mouse leukemia: A model of a multiple-gene disease. *J. Natl. Cancer Inst. 49* (1972): 927.

F. Lilly and R. Steeves. Antigens of murine leukemia viruses. *Biochim. Biophys. Acta 355* (1974): 105.

H. T. Lynch. Cancer and heredity: Implications for early cancer detection. *GP 38* (1968): 78.

H. T. Lynch and A. J. Krush. Differential diagnosis of the cancer family syndrome. *Surgery, Gynecol. Obstetrics 136* (1973): 221.

H. T. Lynch and A. J. Krush. Heredity and adenocarcinoma of the colon. *Gastroenterology 53* (1967): 517.

C. L. Markert. Neoplasia: A disease of cell differentiation. *Cancer Res. 28* (1968): 1908.

C. P. Miles. Non-random chromosome changes in human cancer. *Brit. J. Cancer 30* (1974): 73.

R. W. Miller. Deaths from childhood leukemia and solid tumors, twins and other sibs in the United States, 1960-1967. *J. Natl. Cancer Inst. 46* (1971): 203.

B. Mintz, and K. Illmensee. Normal genetically mosaic mice produced from malignant teratocarcinoma cells. *Proc. Natl. Acad. Sci. USA 72* (1975): 3585.

W. S. Murray and C. C. Little. Genetic studies of carcinogenesis in mice. *J. Natl. Cancer Inst. 38* (1967): 639.

P. C. Nowell. Genetic changes in cancer: Cause or effect? *Human Pathol. 2* (1971): 347.

R. C. Nowinski, E. Fleissner, and N. H. Sarkar. Structural and serological aspects of the oncornaviruses. *Perspect. Virol. 8* (1973): 31.

S. Ohno. Genetic implication of karyological instability of malignant somatic cells. *Physiol. Rev. 51* (1971): 496.

V. E. Papaioannou, M. W. McBurney, and R. L. Gardner. Fate of teratocarcinoma cells injected into early mouse embryos. *Nature 258* (1975): 68.

M. C. Paterson, B. P. Smith, P. H. M. Lohman, A. K. Anderson, and L. Fishman. Defective excision repair of ray-damaged DNA in human (ataxia telangiectasia) fibroblasts. *Nature 260* (1976): 444.

G. B. Pierce. Differentiation of normal and malignant cells. *Fed. Proc. 29* (1970): 1248.

H. C. Pitot. Neoplasia and differentiation as translational functions. In *Developmental Aspects of Carcinogenesis and Immunity* (T.J. King, ed.). Academic, New York, 1974; pp. 79.

P. K. Poon, R. L. O'Brien and J. W. Parker. Defective DNA repair in Fanconi's anemia. *Nature 250* (1974): 223.

P. N. Rosenthal, H. L. Robinson, W. S. Robinson, T. Hanafusa, and H. Hanafusa. DNA in uninfected and virus-infected cells complementary to avian tumor virus RNA. *Proc. Natl. Acad. Sci. USA 68:* (1971): 2336.

W. P. Rowe. Genetic factors in the natural history of murine leukemia virus infection: G. H. A. Clowes Memorial Lecture, *Cancer Res. 33* (1973): 3061.

J. D. Rowley. Do human tumors show a chromosome pattern specific for each etiologic agent? *J. Natl. Cancer Inst. 52* (1974): 315.

J. Schlom, S. Spiegelman, and D. H. Moore. Detection of high molecular weight RNA in particles from human milk. *Science 175* (1972): 542.

E. Stubblefield. The structure of mammalian chromosomes. *Int. Rev. Cytol. 35* (1973): 1.

H. M. Temin. The cellular and molecular biology of RNA tumor viruses, especially avian leukosis-sarcoma viruses and their relatives. *Adv. Cancer Res. 19* (1974): 48.

H. M. Temin and S. Mizutani. RNA-dependent DNA polymerase in virions of Rous sarcoma virus. *Nature 226* (1970): 1211.

M. Terzi. Chromosomal variation and the origin of drug-resistant mutants in mammalian cell lines. *Proc. Natl. Acad. Sci. USA 71* (1974): 5027.

P. K. Vogt. The emerging genetics of RNA tumor viruses. *J. Natl. Cancer Inst. 48* (1972): 3.

B. Watson, T. C. Currier, M. P. Gordon, M. D. Chilton, and E. W. Nester. Plasmid required for virulence of *Agrobacterium tumefaciens. J. Bacteriol. 123* (1975): 255.

S. R. Wolman, T. F. Phillips, and F. F. Becker. Fluorescent banding patterns of rat chromosomes in normal cells and primary hepatocellular carcinomas. *Science 175* (1972): 1267.

T. Yamamoto, Z. Rabinowitz, and L. Sachs. Identification of the chromosomes that control malignancy. *Nature New Biol. 243* (1973): 247.

5

The Etiology
of Human Cancer

Percival Pott initiated the field of chemical carcinogenesis and was one of the
first to study the epidemiology of neoplasia; but, in spite of much work since
then, many questions concerning the etiology of neoplasia in humans are still
unanswered. Furthermore, it is likely that, at least for the foreseeable future,
we will be able to find these answers only through epidemiologic studies.
Clearly no human wishes to be infected by a possible carcinogenic virus in
order to satisfy Koch's postulates, and only a very few have been willing
guinea pigs for the study of chemical carcinogenesis.

Chemical Carcinogens in Human Beings

Materials of Unknown Structure

Table 7 lists a number of materials for which there is reasonably good epidemiologic evidence for a causative relationship to cancer in the human.
The classical findings of Percival Pott on scrotal cancer in the chimney sweep
were one of the first reports of chemical carcinogenesis in humans. Epidermoid carcinoma of the hand, occurring in individuals in the cotton spinning
industry, probably represents a similar relationship between the oils used in
the industry and the genesis of neoplasia in the skin of that part receiving the
highest exposure. Although the exact chemical involved here is unknown, it is
in all likelihood one or more of the polycyclic aromatic hydrocarbons, such
as benzpyrene.

    In the same general category there is strong evidence for a relationship
between smoke from a variety of combustibles and certain types of cancer.

Table 7. Chemical Carcinogens in Humans – Materials in Which the Precise
Chemical Structure of the Etiologic Agent(s) Is Unknown

Material	Associated neoplasm in:
Coke, tar, oils	Skin, scrotum
Iron ore, hematite	Lung
Tobacco smoke	Larynx, bronchus, lung (mouth), bladder
Asbestos	Mesothelium
Wood dust	Nasal cavity and sinuses
Dietary factors	Stomach, colon

In parts of Iceland the very high mortality from gastric cancer is associated
with the high proportion of smoked foods in the diet. The numerous studies
on the composition of tobacco smoke and its effects in experimental animals
amply indicate the relationship between this environmental hazard and cancer
of the respiratory tract.

The association of occupational exposure to asbestos and the subsequent development of bronchogenic carcinoma and mesothelioma has been
well established. However, in virtually all of the studies undertaken in this
field, the highest incidence of both types of neoplasms was found in those individuals exposed to asbestos who also had a history of cigarette smoking.
One study of 17,800 asbestos insulation workers in the United States and
Canada indicated that the risk of bronchogenic carcinoma in nonsmokers who
had been exposed to asbestos was very much lower than in smokers, thus suggesting the probable necessity for multiple environmental agents in the production of lung cancer in individuals exposed to asbestos. On the other hand,
there have been several documented cases of individuals developing mesotheliomas many years after an extremely short exposure to asbestos. Further
evidence in support of the direct carcinogenic effect of asbestos is the fact
that mesotheliomas can be induced in rodents by appropriate exposure to
this material. However, although other fibrous materials such as fiberglass
have been shown to be carcinogenic in the rodent, there is essentially no evidence to date that fibrous glass causes human cancer. Although the mechanism of asbestos induction of cancer is as yet unknown, the demonstration
of the importance of fiber size to the carcinogenicity of this material suggests
that its carcinogenic action may not be too dissimilar to that of the "plastic
film" carcinogenesis, which we had discussed earlier. On the other hand, there
is essentially no epidemiologic evidence at present for the occurrence of
plastic film carcinogenesis in humans as it is seen in experimental animals.

A situation similar to the problem of asbestos exposure may be seen in underground hematite miners in several areas of Europe as well as in this country. Since iron oxide has not been found to be carcinogenic in laboratory animals, although hematite dust enhances the carcinogenic activity of hydrocarbons in the lung, the exact agent or agents producing the increased incidence of lung cancer in this occupational group has not yet been identified. Similarly, workers in the furniture industry and related fields exposed to high levels of wood dust are prone to adenocarcinoma of the nasal cavity and sinuses. A similar finding has been demonstrated in workers in the shoe industry in England. Again the exact offending agent is unknown.

Among those agents influencing the incidence of cancer in human beings as evidenced from epidemiologic studies, the role of diet in the production of stomach and colon cancer has become one of the most recent concerns of oncologists. As mentioned above, the relatively high incidence of gastric cancer in Iceland can be statistically related to the high level of smoked fish consumed in that country. But as yet the dietary factors involved in the high morbidity and mortality rates of stomach cancer in Japan have not been identified. In this country the suggestion has been made that one reason for the decrease in gastric cancer seen over the past 2 or 3 decades is the addition of antioxidants to dairy products and other foods containing fat. However, this proposal has never been adequately verified. While the dietary control of atherosclerosis is presently a popular medical regimen, some evidence indicates that a high consumption of fats and oils is also related to an increased incidence of malignant neoplasms of the breast, ovaries, and rectum. After initial suggestive data for a positive correlation, further study has not implicated polyunsaturated fatty acid diets in colon cancer, although in a retrospective study a majority of patients with colon cancer were found to have relatively low serum cholesterol levels. Recent epidemiologic studies of cancer of the colon have demonstrated its high frequency in this country and its relative absence in certain parts of Africa. Dietary factors have been suggested as playing a primary role in the differential incidence of this disease. The bulky diet of certain African native populations, where cancer of the colon and rectum is relatively rare, has been suggested as one primary factor in the low incidence of this disease in these populations. On the other hand, some investigators have suggested that differences in the bacterial flora of the two populations may be of major pathogenetic significance. More recent evidence suggests that meat, particularly beef, is one foodstuff associated with the development of malignancies of the large bowel.

Naturally Occurring Carcinogenic Chemicals

One class of naturally occurring chemical carcinogens (Table 8) for which there is reasonable epidemiologic evidence for their existence as a causative factor in human cancer is that of the mold toxins, especially aflatoxin B_1. The importance of the mold toxin aflatoxin in relation to liver cancer in certain parts of Africa, especially Kenya and Uganda, has now been reasonably documented. In more than one study an association has been made between the aflatoxin content of food and the frequency of hepatomas. While in this country aflatoxin ingestion is not considered to be a problem since foodstuffs likely to contain the toxin, such as peanut butter, are carefully monitored for its content, still there has been at least one documented case of cancer of the liver in a U.S. resident associated with high levels of aflatoxin B_1 in this organ. While other mold toxins such as sterigmatocystin have been suggested as additional etiologic factors in human liver cancer, the evidence for their role in this disease in not as convincing at the present time.

Other natural products such as the pyrrolizidine alkaloids, which occur in extracts of various roots found in the West Indies and other parts of the world, cycasin obtained from extracts of the cycad nut, and safrole, a naturally occurring seasoning agent, have been shown to be carcinogenic for the liver in rodents. As yet there is no significant evidence that these materials cause hepatomas in humans although the pyrrolizidine alkaloids have been implicated in the production of vascular disease of the liver in Jamaica and other West Indian countries.

Table 8. Chemical Carcinogens in Humans — Naturally Occurring Chemical Carcinogens

Chemical	Associated neoplasm in:
Aflatoxin B_1 (sterigmatocystin?)	Liver
Nickel	Lung, nasal sinuses
Cadmium	Lung, prostate
Chromates	Lung
Arsenic	Skin

Industrial hazards related to naturally occurring chemical carcinogens are seen predominantly in the metal industry. Nickel, usually in the form of nickel carbonyl, a chemical produced during the refining of the ore, has been implicated on the basis of epidemiologic and clinical investigations as a causative agent in cancer of the lung and nasal sinuses among workers. Similarly, workers in the production of cadmium and also of various chromium compounds, especially pigments, have been shown to suffer from increased incidences of prostatic malignancies and pulmonary cancer, respectively. One of the more interesting elemental carcinogens is arsenic, which appears to be carcinogenic for the skin of humans when it is taken internally for long periods of time. As yet arsenic administration to animal species other than humans has not resulted in the production of neoplasia.

Synthetic Chemical Carcinogens

It has been estimated that tens of thousands of new, previously unknown chemicals enter our environment through industry and research every year. The carcinogenic potential of the vast majority of these compounds will probably never be known unless newer methodologies for carcinogen testing are discovered.

Table 9 lists some of the more important chemicals that have been shown with reasonable certainty to be carcinogenic in human beings. The most significant of this group are those related to industry. Recently, because of overwhelming evidence for the importance of a number of these chemicals as causative factors in human neoplasia, a total of 14 specific chemicals, not all of which are listed in the table, have been termed by law in this country as carcinogenic hazards for the human, and special precautions must be utilized in handling these compounds. In addition to those compounds listed, the following compounds are also defined as carcinogens: 2-acetylaminofluorene, 3,3'-dichlorobenzidine, 4-dimethylaminoazobenzene, α-naphthylamine, β-propiolactone, bis-chloromethyl ether, 4,4'-methylene (bis)-2-chloroaniline, and ethyleneimine.

The importance of the aromatic amines as etiologic agents in cancer of the bladder is well known. Although the studies of mustard gas are less well known, there is substantial evidence to implicate this compound as a pulmonary carcinogen in humans. Recent evidence of the importance of vinyl chloride in the production of angiosarcomas in the liver of humans has been reasonably well documented.

Table 9. Chemical Carcinogens in Humans — Synthetic (Man-Made) Chemical Carcinogens

Chemicals	Associated neoplasm in:
Industry	
2-naphthylamine, benzidine, 4-amino biphenyl, 4 nitro biphenyl	Bladder
Bis(2-chloroethyl) sulfide	Lung
Chloromethyl methyl ether	Lung
Vinyl chloride	Liver (angiosarcoma)
Drugs	
Phenacetin	Renal pelvis
Immunosuppressive drugs	Lymphoma
Cyclophosphamide, melphalan	Bladder (leukemia?)
Chloramphenicol	Leukemia?
Estrogen therapy, premenopausal	Liver (adenomas predominantly), uterus
Estrogen therapy, postmenopausal	Uterus
Androgens	Liver
Food additives	
Nitrite (+ amines) (nitrosamines)	Esophagus? colon?

The extensive use of new drugs in the therapy of human disease has not been without complications. The list of drugs shown to be carcinogenic in the human is supported by a reasonable degree of evidence. However, in many instances, the mechanism appears to be complicated. The association of carcinoma of the renal pelvis with phenacetin is most prevalent in Europe, where this compound is prescribed quite routinely and in large doses for prolonged periods. A number of immunosuppressive drugs, including imuran, prednisone, and others, have been implicated as carcinogens because of the relatively high incidence of lymphomas found in patients with transplants. However, it is not clear whether these compounds actually are carcinogenic themselves or act by suppressing the natural resistance of the host to malignant cells already present. On the other hand, the alkylating agents, cyclophosphamide and melphalan, have been implicated in bladder carcinoma in young children treated earlier in life for acute leukemia. This is being seen only now with the exceedingly long survival produced in a significant number of cases of childhood leukemia.

The effect of estrogen administration to pregnant women on the genesis of malignant uterine and vaginal cancer in the offspring is now well documented, as we have discussed previously. As further evidence of the carcinogenicity of some estrogenic preparations, recent findings have demonstrated the association of liver cell adenomas with the relatively prolonged use of oral contraceptives containing synthetic estrogens. In addition, in at least one instance carcinoma of the endometrium also occurred following long-term sequential oral contraception. Very recently several retrospective studies have also demonstrated that menopausal and postmenopausal women given estrogens have a higher incidence of uterine cancer than those not treated with this hormone. Prior to all of these findings, a number of reports had demonstrated that androgen therapy was associated with hepatomas. Thus sex hormones do appear to be potentially, if not actually, carcinogenic for the human under certain physiologic conditions of age, sex, etc.

Despite the legislation in the early part of this century to prohibit the addition of known carcinogens to foodstuffs in the diet of the American citizen, potential carcinogenic chemicals still remain in the diet largely because of our own ignorance. The example cited in Table 9 has not been eliminated as a food additive in this country. Although nitrites themselves are not carcinogenic, they can react with amines both in the food and in the intestine to produce carcinogenic nitrosamines. The finding of dimethylnitrosamine in fish meal treated with nitrite and the presence in flour of diethylnitrosamine, produced from drying the grain in a stream of exhaust gases containing oxides of nitrogen, are ample evidence that such compounds can be produced. Furthermore, experimental studies have shown the production of a number of different malignancies of the gastrointestinal tract by the addition of nitrite and amines to the diet.

The FDA has been very reluctant in the past few years to allow additions to our diet even if the evidence for carcinogenicity is quite remote. An excellent example of this is the controversy over the artificial sweetener, cyclamate. In addition. while not strictly a food additive, the administration of diethylstilbestrol to cattle in order to increase the yield of their meat has been declared to be potentially hazardous for consumers of beef. As yet, however, because of legal complications no definitive action has been taken to regulate the addition of this agent indirectly to the American diet.

Methods for Obtaining Data Supporting the Carcinogenicity of Chemicals in Humans

A number of techniques have been utilized to determine the potential carcinogenic risk of chemicals and materials present in our environment. The principles involved in these studies involve statistics and careful observation. The following are some of the general means of obtaining epidemiologic data:

1. *Episodic observations.* The observation of isolated cases of cancer in relation to a specific environmental factor has been used in the past to afford clues to a cause-and-effect relationship. However, in many instances careful statistical evaluation of the data shows that it can be very misleading, and the usefulness of such observations is presently open to question, at least as a general method for obtaining significant data.

2. *Retrospective studies.* Investigations after the fact and later development of disease in a group of individuals have been used quite frequently as a method of obtaining epidemiologic data. A very important factor in such investigations is the use of case controls, and in many instances the suitable designation of such controls is the critical component in the study. In general, this type of study is usually the first step in attempting to identify causative factors.

3. *Prospective studies.* These investigations involve analyses of the development of individuals with specific social habits, occupational exposures, etc. Such investigations require large populations, long follow-up periods (5-20 years), and high follow-up rates for both controls and test groups. Many such investigations are presently under way in this country and throughout the world.

4. *Multifactorial studies.* In general, factors that lead to cancer in humans are quite probably multifactorial in a large number of instances. Such factors include chemicals, radiation, genetic background, and biological agents, and may be additive, synergistic, or antagonistic. Several agents may act at the same stage (such as initiation or promotion) or at different stages. Thus such studies are complicated and require the evaluation of several variables.

Epidemiologic studies can only identify factors that are different between two populations and that are sufficiently important in the etiology of the condition under study to play a determining role under the conditions of exposure. On the other side of the coin, knowledge from basic investigations can be extremely helpful in prospective multifactorial studies of human populations. One of the most important thrusts of research affecting epidemiologic studies in humans is the search for a rapid and foolproof method of identifying carcinogenic chemicals and compounds. While any such system, unless involving the human directly, is open to the criticism that a material carcinogenic for one species or in one system may not be carcinogenic in another, still such studies are extremely important in order to identify potential hazards in the human environment.

The principal methods used to establish the carcinogenicity of environmental factors are several:

1. *Animal studies.* These are tedious and expensive but in the last analysis are the only method to establish the carcinogenic potential of a suspected compound. Such investigations involve feeding or administering suspected carcinogens to various animal populations and watching for the development of neoplasms over extended periods of time (months and years).

2. *In vitro transformation of cells in culture.* This relatively new tool offers promise to identify chemicals that can cause the malignant transformation or related phenomena in cells grown in culture. has the advantage of rapidity but the disadvantage that not all transformed cells exhibit biological neoplasia in vivo. Furthermore, although human tissues in culture may be used directly as test agents, the known metabolic activation which must occur for many compounds to become carcinogenic does not occur in most tissues easily cultured in vitro.

3. *Microsomal-bacterial mutagenic systems.* One of the most recent and most promising methods for the rapid establishment of the carcinogenicity of chemicals is the use of liver microsome systems, which are incubated with the suspected carcinogenic agent, and the incubation mix subsequently added to a highly mutable bacterium or directly to transforming DNA. This system and its effectiveness in scoring human carcinogens have been extensively studied by Ames and his associates. The incidences of specific types of mutations are then scored and related to the metabolic conversion of the

original agent and the ability of such metabolites to induce mutations. Thus far the correlation between agents mutagenic in this
system and their carcinogenicity in vivo is quite good. However, a
few agents that are unlikely or not known to be mutagenic (e.g.,
asbestos, plastic film, and others) would not be picked up by this
system.

Finally in obtaining epidemiological data it is important that when a
suspected compound or chemical is studied, the effect would be expected to
show a dose-response relationship. Such an effect is easily measured in experimental animal systems, but becomes quite difficult in human studies.

Viral Carcinogenesis in Humans

A major question in the etiology of human neoplasia is whether or not viruses
are important in the causation of human cancer. Literally millions of dollars
have been spent in this country trying to answer this particular question. However, the best evidence for such a relationship emanated from some observations by a practicing English physician in central Africa, Dr. Dennis Burkitt.
Dr. Burkitt noted the occurrence of a peculiar type of lymphoma in children
in certain areas of the African continent. The tumors occurred only in individuals living above a certain altitude and in certain climatic areas. This indicated to Burkitt a possible insect vector in the disease, and he suggested that
a virus was the causative agent. Within a relatively few years, Burkitt's hypothesis was supported in that a virus was isolated from patients with the lymphoma that now bears his name. The virus isolated, the EB virus, is a member
of the herpes group of viruses.
    There is now substantial evidence for a close association, if not a causal
relationship, between the EB virus and two neoplasms in the human being.
The Burkitt lymphoma, which occurs almost exclusively in certain areas of
central Africa, is ubiquitously associated with the EB virus, which can be isolated or demonstrated by techniques of molecular biology in all patients with
this disease. Such is not the case in the United States, where Burkitt's lymphoma is only infrequently associated with the EB virus. In addition, a very
high frequency of association occurs between the EB virus and nasopharyngeal
carcinoma in areas of the Far East, particularly southern China. In this instance,
as with Burkitt's lymphoma, the virus has been demonstrated directly within
the nuclei of the neoplastic cells. In addition to the presence of the virus in
these two neoplastic conditions in humans, this virus has also been associated with at least two nonneoplastic conditions, sarcoidosis and infectious

mononucleosis. This latter disease has been shown to be infectious in the human, and recently the causative agent has been identified as the EB virus. Most individuals in the American population have antibodies to the EB virus and thus are resistant to "reinfection." The major problem is how this virus can cause a relatively innocuous disease in individuals in this nation and also apparently cause malignant disease in populations in other parts of the world.

Recent evidence has suggested that the herpes simplex 2 virus may be associated with human cervical cancer, but there is no reproducible evidence as yet for this association. Also some recent biochemical evidence has indicated the possible existence in human milk of particles indistinguishable from certain animal viruses, some of which are oncogenic, namely the C-type viruses and the mammary tumor virus. The evidence for this is both structural, from the electron microscope, and also biochemical, in that a 70S RNA and reverse transcriptase activity were demonstrated within human breast tumors and human milk.

Papovaviruses have been isolated from the tissues of patients afflicted with a relatively rare disease of the central nervous system, progressive multifocal leucoencephalopathy (PML). Initially the virus was isolated from brain tissue obtained at autopsy from a case of PML complicating Hodgkin's disease. This virus was grown in human fetal glial cells and has been termed the JC virus. In addition, another papovavirus termed the BK virus has been isolated from the urine of a patient who had been immunosuppressed for several months. Neither of these viruses has much antigenic relationship to other primate or murine papovaviruses. However, viruses resembling SV40 have been isolated from the brains of two patients with PML. These latter viruses are antigenically quite similar to SV40, and both JC and BK viruses exhibit some cross-reactivity of their T antigens with that of the SV40 virus. In rodents both the BK virus and the JC virus are capable of inducing neoplasms. In addition, there is similar evidence for the oncogenicity in lower animals of a common human pathogen, the cytomegalovirus, which is a herpesvirus. However, evidence for its direct oncogenicity in human beings has not yet been reported.

Thus, with the exception of the EB virus, there is at present no known oncogenic human virus, either DNA or RNA, although recent epidemiologic evidence has strongly indicated an association of hepatitis B virus with hepatomas in African patients. In view of the intensive search presently going on, if such a virus does exist, it should come to light within the next decade.

References

M. E. Alpert, M. S. R. Hutt, G. N. Wogan, and C. S. Davidson. Association between aflatoxin content of food and hepatoma frequency in Uganda. *Cancer 28* (1971): 253.

R. Axel, S. C. Gulati, and S. Spiegelman. Particles containing RNA-instructed DNA polymerase and virus-related RNA in human breast cancers. *Proc. Natl. Acad. Sci. USA 69* (1972): 3133.

H. R. Bierman. Predictive oncology. *Int. Surg. 58* (1973): 683 and 763.

B. S. Blumberg, B. Larouze, W. Thomas, B. Werner, J. E. Hesser, I. Millman, G. Saimot, and M. Payet. The relation of infection with the hepatitis B agent to primary hepatic carcinoma. *Am. J. Pathol. 81* (1975): 669.

P. Brodeur. Annals of industry (industrial casualties, I-V), *The New Yorker,* October 29-November 26, 1973. An informed lay report – with emphasis on episodic reporting.

R. Doll and I. Vodopija (eds.). Host environment interactions in the etiology of cancer in man. International Agency for Research on Cancer, Lyon, 1973.

R. Doll, L. G. Morgan, and F. E. Speizer. Cancers of the lung and nasal sinuses in nickel workers. *Brit. J. Cancer 24* (1970): 623.

H. A. Edmondson, B. Henderson, and B. Benton. Liver-cell adenomas associated with the use of oral contraceptives. *New Eng. J. Med. 294* (1976): 470.

W. G. Figuerpa, R. Paszkowski, and W. Weiss. Lung cancer in chloromethyl methyl ether workers. *N. Eng. J. Med. 288* (1973): 1096.

J. F. Fraumeni (ed.). *Persons at High Risk of Cancer – An Approach to Cancer Etiology and Control.* Academic, New York, 1975.

J. F. Fraumeni. Respiratory carcinogenesis: An epidemiologic appraisal. *J. Natl. Cancer Inst. 55* (1975): 1039.

J. F. Fraumeni and R. W. Miller. Drug-induced cancer. *J. Natl. Cancer Inst. 48* (1972): 1267.

S. Goldfarb. Sex hormones and hepatic neoplasia. *Cancer Res. 36* (1976): 2584.

S. Heyden. Polyunsaturated fatty acids and colon cancer. *Nutr. Metabol. 17* (1974): 321.

J. Higginson. Present trends in cancer epidemiology. *Can. Cancer Conf. 8* (1969): 40.

J. Higginson and C. S. Muir. Epidemiology. In *Cancer Medicine* (J. F. Holland and E. Frei, eds.). Lea and Fibiger, Philadelphia, 1973, p. 241.

M. A. Howell. Diet as an etiological factor in the development of cancers of the colon and rectum. *J. Chron. Dis. 28* (1975): 67.

M. D. Innis. Burkitt's lymphoma and heredity. *Oncology 28* (1973): 184.

J. H. Joncas. Clinical significance of the EB herpes virus infection in man. *Prog. Med. Virol 14* (1972): 200.

L. G. Koss, M. R. Melamed, and R. E. Kelly. Further cytologic and histologic studies of bladder lesions in workers exposed to para-aminodiphenyl: Progress report. *J. Natl. Cancer Inst. 43* (1969): 233.

S. Langard and T. Norseth. A cohort study of bronchial carcinomas in workers producing chromate pigments. *Brit. J. Indust. Med. 32* (1975): 62.

A. M. Lilienfeld, M. L. Levin, and I. I. Kessler. *Cancer in the United States.* Harvard University Press, Cambridge, 1972.

F. A. Lyon. The development of adenocarcinoma of the endometrium in young women receiving long-term sequential oral contraception. *Am. J. Obstet. Gynecol. 123* (1975): 299.

T. M. Mack, M. C. Pike, B. E. Henderson, R. I. Pfeffer, V. R. Gerkins, M. Arthur, and S. E. Brown. Estrogens and endometrial cancer in a retirement community. *New Eng. J. Med. 294* (1976): 1262.

T. W. Mak, S. Kurtz, J. Manaster, and D. Housman. Viral-related information in oncornavirus-like particles isolated from cultures of marrow cells from leukemic patients in relapse and remission. *Proc. Natl. Acad. Sci. USA 72* (1975): 623.

R. J. Mangi, J. C. Niederman, J. E. Kelleher, J. M. Dwyer, A. S. Evans, and F. S. Kantor. Depression of cell-mediated immunity during acute infectious mononucleosis. *New Eng. J. Med. 291* (1974): 1149.

J. McCann and B. N. Ames. Detection of carcinogens as mutagens in the *Salmonella*/microsome test: Assay of 300 chemicals: Discussion. *Proc. Natl. Acad. Sci. USA 73* (1976): 950.

A. T. Meadows, J. L. Naiman, and M. Valdes-Dapena. Hepatoma associated with androgen therapy for aplastic anemia. *J. Peds. 84* (1974): 109.

J. Milne. Are glass fibres carcinogenic to man? A critical appraisal. *Brit. J. Indust. Med. 33* (1976): 47.

C. Moore. Cigarette smoking and cancer of the mouth, pharynx and larynx. *J. Am. Med. Assoc. 218* (1971): 553.

W. Nakahara, T. Hirayama, K. Nishioka, and H. Sugano (eds.). *Analytical and Experimental Epidemiology of Cancer.* University Park Press, Baltimore, 1973.

M. Nonoyama and J. S. Pagano. Homology between Epstein-Barr virus DNA and viral DNA from Burkitt's lymphoma and nasopharyngeal carcinoma determined by DNA-RNA reassociation kinetics. *Nature 242* (1973): 44.

R. Oyasu and M. L. Hopp. The etiology of cancer of the bladder. *Surg. Gynecol Obs. 138* (1974): 97.

F. G. Peers and C. A. Linsell. Aflatoxins and liver cancer – a population-based study in Kenya. *Brit. J. Cancer 27* (1973): 473.

D. L. Phillips, D. M. Yourtee, and S. Searles. Presence of aflatoxin B_1 in human liver in the United States. *Tox. Appl. Pharmacol. 36* (1976): 403.

F. J. C. Roe. Carcinogenesis and sanity. *Fd. Cosmet. Toxicol. 6* (1968): 485.

U. Saffiotti and J. K. Wagoner (eds.). Occupational carcinogenesis. *N. Y. Acad. Sci. 271* (1976): 1.

T. Shope, D. Dechairo, and G. Miller. Malignant lymphoma in cotton top marmosets after inoculation with Epstein-Barr virus. *Proc. Natl. Acad. Sci. USA 70* (1973): 2487.

R. T. Smith and J. C. Bausber. Epstein-Barr virus infection in relation to infectious mononucleosis and Burkitt's lymphoma. *Ann. Rev. Med. 23* (1972): 39.

Smoking and health. Report of the Advisory Committee to the Surgeon General of the Public Health Service, USPHS, Publ. 1103, 1964.

M. F. Stanton. Fiber carcinogenesis: Is asbestos the only hazard? *J. Natl. Cancer Inst. 52* (1974): 633.

S. Wada, M. Miyanishi, Y. Nishimoto, S. Kambe, and R. W. Miller. Mustard gas as a cause of respiratory neoplasia in man. *Lancet 1* (1968): 1161.

J. C. Wagner. Asbestos cancers. *J. Natl. Cancer Inst. 46* (1971): v.

L. P. Weiner, and O. Narayan. Virologic studies of progressive multifocal Leukoencephalopathy. *Prog. Med. Virol. 18* (1974): 229.

S. Yeh. Skin cancer in chronic arsenicism. *Human Pathol. 4* (1973): 469.

6

The Pathogenesis of Cancer

The Latency of Neoplasia

One of the ubiquitous characteristics of carcinogenesis in vivo is the occurrence of an extended period of time between the initial application of a carcinogen — be it physical, chemical, or biological — and the appearance of a neoplasm. Several workers, including Rous, Berenblum, and others, suggested more than 20 years ago that carcinogenesis may be divided into at least two stages: the stage of *initiation*, resulting from the application of a carcinogen directly to a cellular population, and the stage of *promotion*, which occurs subsequent to initiation and results from environmental factors, principally the application of so-called "cocarcinogenic" compounds. The basic experimental protocol utilized by Berenblum and others is depicted in Figure 13. Most studies have demonstrated that the process of initiation is essentially irreversible, although applications of small doses of carcinogens to the skin of mice may not be followed by neoplasms unless a cocarcinogen is applied thereafter. Studies by Boutwell, Berenblum, Shubik and others demonstrated that when the application of the cocarcinogen is delayed for 9 to 12 months in the mouse, neoplasms will still result even after this delayed interrval. Recently, studies by Roe and his associates have indicated that a year's delay between initiation and the application of the promoting agent results in very few or no tumors; this would seem to indicate that under some circumstances initiation may be "reversible." In contrast to the relatively stable initiated state, promotion may be modified by a number of environmental factors, including diet, age, sex, hormonal balance, etc. Some experimental investigations have indicated that promotion may be reversed.

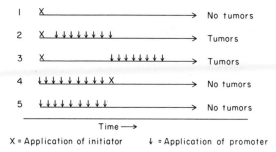

Time ⟶

X = Application of initiator   ↓ = Application of promoter

Figure 13. Outline of the scheme of initiation and promotion developed from studies of carcinogenesis in mouse skin. Each line represents an experimental condition in which there is no or a single application of the initiating agent, usually a carcinogenic polycyclic hydrocarbon at a subcarcinogenic dose. The multiple arrows represent multiple applications of the promoting agent, croton oil, phorbol ester, or other known promoter for mouse skin. The time span may extend from 15 to 50 weeks, depending on dosages of the initiator and promoter utilized and the mouse strain employed in the experiment. The term "tumors" refers to papillomas or to carcinomas, provided the experiment is extended for a sufficiently long time.

Although the two-stage mechanism of carcinogenesis has been almost totally established in and applied to epidermal carcinogenesis, other analogous examples have been demonstrated. In the case of radiation-induced hepatomas, we have already seen that partial hepatectomy or administration of carbon tetrachloride will "promote" the formation of many more tumors than is possible by radiation alone. In this instance, the neutrons or γ rays are the initiating agent, whereas the proliferative stimulus is the promoter. Another interesting example of the two-stage phenomenon of carcinogenesis is that of the chemical induction of bladder cancer by N-methyl-N-nitrosourea (MNU). The protocol for this experiment is seen in Figure 14A and is quite analogous to that described for the skin except that the promotor or co-carcinogen, saccharin, is fed for 6 weeks prior to and 48 weeks following a single administration of 2 mg of MNU directly into the bladder or rats. MNU administration or saccharin feeding alone produce moderate to slight hyperplasia of the bladder epithelium, respectively, but no carcinomas. The experiment strongly suggests that in order for bladder cancer to occur as the result of the administration of this carcinogen, the target cell in the bladder epithelium must be stimulated either by further administration of MNU or by a promoting agent such as saccharin. Under the circumstances of this experiment,

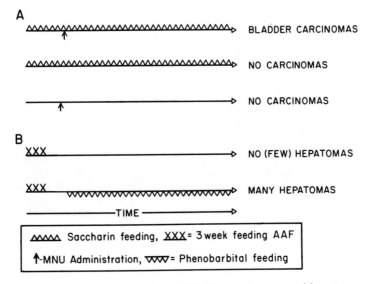

Figure 14. Initiation and promotion of bladder carcinomas and hepatomas. The initiating agents are noted in the figure. The time span represented is up to 13 months for MNU and 6 months for AAF.

saccharin did not act as a carcinogen as has been claimed as a result of some recent experiments; this led to a public furor because of the potential removal of this material from the market in the United States.

In the case of the skin it has been possible to distinguish between agents that have essentially only a promoting action and thus are truly termed cocarcinogens and those that are capable of both initiation and promotion and thus are termed complete carcinogens. In addition, some agents such as urethan, when given systemically, will initiate skin cells which in the absence of a promoting agent will never exhibit their neoplastic potential. On the other hand, after systemic initiation by urethan, carcinoma of the skin will occur after promotion with known cocarcinogens such as croton oil in the protocol as described in Figure 13. Thus urethan and agents with similar actions may be termed "pure" initiators for the skin. In the human, evidence has accumulated for the existence of tumor-promoting fractions in cigarette smoke; the evidence indicates that lung carcinogenesis may be the result of both tumor initiation and tumor promotion, the latter possibly acting on cells initiated by as yet unknown materials.

Recently an entirely new system, which is completely analogous to that seen in the skin, has been reported by Peraino and his associates to occur in hepatocarcinogenesis. In this system the potent hepatocarcinogen, acetylaminofluorene, is fed in very small doses for short periods of time to rats. After only 3 weeks of feeding, the carcinogen is removed from the diet, and the animals are maintained on standard laboratory chow. Very few neoplasms result wit023 the next 6 months. However, if phenobarbital is added to the diet after the carcinogen is removed, then within 6 months almost 100% of the animals exhibit hepatic neoplasms. This protocol is outlined in Figure 14B. This system not only demonstrates that initiation and promotion may be elicited in organs other than skin, but it also presents the difficult problem that many components in our environment that are not carcinogenic may lead to promotion of neoplasms in many different organs. Furthermore, it is quite possible that promotion by such compounds as phenobarbital may bring out and magnify the effects of very weak carcinogens that occur in the human diet or in other environmental situations.

The exact mechanism of action of cocarcinogens is not yet clear. As indicated above, hyperplasia during cocarcinogenesis certainly plays a major role. Experiments on carcinogenesis in vitro have indicated that cells must undergo at least one cell division in the presence of the carcinogen in order for the neoplastic transformation to be "fixed" into the transformed cell. More recent studies have indicated that a number of cocarcinogens are potent inhibitors of DNA repair, but this does not appear to be an effect specific for such compounds. The purification and determination of structure of the principal cocarcinogenic constituents of croton oil, the most popular cocarcinogen used in the mouse skin system, have opened the doorway to a much more exact definition of the biochemical changes occurring in cells during both initiation and promotion.

The two-stage concept of carcinogenesis has important applications for human cancer. It is obvious that at the present time the average human being living in a city comes in contact with numerous carcinogenic compounds throughout his life. Since it is apparent that relatively small amounts of such compounds are required for initiation, it is possible that some cells within each individual are initiated. However, it is only after a long period of promotion by the same or other chemicals or perhaps by environmental or even hereditary factors that the neoplasm will appear. In support of the two-stage concept in humans is the presence of certain lesions that appear to be the counterpart of the initiated cell. The disease *leukoplakia,* which is an atypical proliferation of mucous epithelium, is a lesion that, if left alone, will in many cases become malignant. There also occurs in the human female breast atypical lobules which may later become associated with a higher frequency of malignant neoplasia than is seen in breasts that contain no atypical lobules. The histologic characteristics of these lobules are quite similar to the hyperplastic alveolar nodules seen in mice. Such lesions in the mouse are clearly preneoplastic, from which frank malignant neoplasms of the breast may arise on continued growth or transplantation. In the human there are also several examples of neoplasms which in themselves are behavioristically benign, but which exhibit a number of characteristics of malignant neoplasms. When these are epithelial in nature, they are called carcinomas in situ. The most common example of carcinoma in situ is seen in the human cervix when a highly anaplastic growth is seen within the confines of the cervical epithelium. The lesion does not invade through the basement membrane and, thus, may be considered as remaining within its normal confines. Carcinoma in situ of the cervix normally occurs in women between ages 30 and 40, whereas invasive, frankly malignant, cervical carcinoma usually occurs after age 40. This definitely indicates a time relationship·between the two and fits into the two-stage theory quite well. Other examples of carcinoma in situ occur in the male prostate as well as in certain types of gastrointestinal adenomas.

The Progression of Neoplasia

Inherent in the concept of the two-stage theory of carcinogenesis is a transition from the initiated cell to the biologically malignant cell. The case of the presumed conversion of carcinoma in situ of the cervix to frankly invasive malignant carcinoma is perhaps an excellent example in the human. However, it is well known that some neoplasms may progress from a very low degree of malignancy to a very rapidly growing virulent and rapidly fatal neoplasm. All of these processes, but more so the latter, have been termed the progression of neoplasia.

This process of progression from a low grade to a high grade of malignancy, or even of a benign to a malignant neoplasm, involves alteration in biological activity as well as in morphologic appearance. The mechanism for this process has been disputed over the years. Basically two mechanisms have been considered, the first being a frank transformation of a whole population of cells from one form to the other. In light of present knowledge, this particular mechanism appears unlikely. On the other hand, the more attractive mechanism and the one presumed to be the major factor in tumor progression is the selection of minority cell types in the low grade or benign neoplasm which then, because of their capability to grow more rapidly or to metabolize at a faster rate, have become the predominant cell type of the population. In many instances this involves a change in karyotype. Evidence for this mechanism of progression is best exemplified during tumor transplantation for many generations. An example of this change in karyotype may be seen in Figure 15, which depicts the normal karyotype (a) of a sarcoma induced in a mouse by the Rous virus. Subsequent transplant generations of this same neoplasm exhibit aneuploid karyotypes (b, c, and d). In most instances, repeated transplantation results in more rapidly growing tumors with a higher degree of aneuploidy. We will again consider the role of progression in the natural history of neoplasia in Chapter 8.

An interesting potential mechanism of progression has recently been suggested by Goldenberg and his associates. They have proposed on the basis of some experimental evidence that hybridization of normal and neoplastic cells may occur in vivo and that this may be an important mechanism in the progression of neoplasms. Their studies, based on karyotypic and morphologic investigations of cells hybridized in vitro and presumably in vivo, lend credence to this potential mechanism of tumor progression, but further investigation must be carried out in order to determine whether such a mechanism is applicable to the vast majority of human and experimental neoplasms.

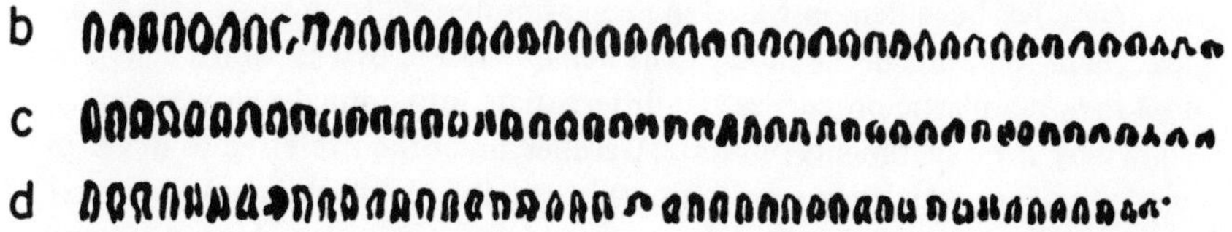

Figure 15. Karyotypes of several transplant generations of a sarcoma in mice induced by the Rous sarcoma virus. Karyotype (a) is that of the primary neoplasm and exhibits an essentially normal appearance and number (40) of chromosomes. Karyotypes (b), (c), and (d) are those of later transplant generations, which have accumulated extra chromosomes as well as abnormal chromosomes. This series demonstrates the karyotypic progression of a neoplasm. (After Mark.)

The Regression of Neoplasia

The fact that neoplasms may regress has been known by experimental oncologists for some years. This can easily be shown in the case of tumors
transplanted into new hosts. The obvious mechanism in this case is that the
host recognizes the tumor as a foreign tissue and, thus, tends to reject it
immunologically. In the human being, examples of tumor regression are quite
rare. It was felt that such examples could also be explained on the basis of
host immunity to the tumor, although in some instances such a mechanism
may not explain the peculiar reaction of the neoplasm. This is particularly
true when certain types of tumors appear to differentiate into adult benign
tissues after initially demonstrating biological malignancy. The mechanism
for this phenomenon has not yet been explained, but it is unlikely that a
mutational mechanism is responsible. Rather, this finding of the differentiation of a malignant neoplasm to benign or even normal tissue is quite compatible with the concept that neoplasia is basically a disease of differentiation.

Perhaps the best-studied example of a "controlled" reversion or differentiation of a neoplasm to a normal cell is seen in the plant. Both the crown
gall tumors briefly discussed earlier and several other plant neoplasms including a teratoma can, under controlled conditions, differentiate and produce a
perfectly normal plant. However, recent studies have demonstrated that the
normal differentiation of neoplastic plant cells occurs without the loss of the
plasmid (see Chapter 4), and thus under appropriate conditions, such as those
seen in cell culture, these cells will again express their biological neoplasia. In
animals, carcinogen-induced epidermoid carcinoma in amphibians will also
differentiate and ultimately disappear from the organism. In the mouse, teratomas may be produced or occur spontaneously. A small percentage of these
neoplasms differentiate into essentially normal tissue types. This latter phenomenon has been demonstrated in neoplasms derived from single cells of a
malignant teratoma in the mouse. The demonstration that teratoma cells will
lose their neoplastic properties and differentiate into normal cells was clearly
shown by the experiments of Mintz, Gardner, and others referred to in Chapter 4. In the human, the neuroblastoma of childhood, which in most cases is
highly malignant and is derived from neuroblasts of the adrenal medulla, may
in a small percentage of cases spontaneously differentiate to a benign ganglio-
neuroma. This latter lesion is a mass of fully differentiated neurons with no
malignant potential remaining. Differentiation of primary cultures of neuroblastoma to normal tissue has also been shown to occur.

Recent studies on cells transformed in vitro have also implied that such
transformed cells may exhibit relatively high rates of "reversion" of their

transformed properties acquired in vitro. The revertants usually are polyploid. In addition, some experiments have demonstrated that somatic cell hybridization of a normal with a malignant cell may result in a cell with "normal" properties. Unfortunately, similar experiments in several laboratories have given variable results, so that the exact conclusions to be drawn from hybridization of normal and malignant cells are not clear at this time.

A number of rather common neoplasms in the human have been shown to regress, sometimes spontaneously. Among these are tumors of the breast, an occasional ovarian carcinoma, and melanomas. With carcinoma of the breast, because of its propensity to remain dormant for some years, the actual phenomenon of regression may be related to several factors. An interesting phenomenon has been described with renal cell carcinomas in that removal of the primary tumor may lead to disappearance of pulmonary metastases. In the special case of the chorioepithelioma, a malignant neoplasm of the placenta, spontaneous regression may be accounted for by host immunity, since the tumor tissue is actually foreign to the maternal immune system. In the male, a morphologically similar neoplasm may arise from host tissues and does not regress spontaneously.

Latent or Occult Carcinoma

The fact that certain neoplasms may remain in the organism for many years without expressing their behavioristic malignancy to any significant degree has been known to clinicians for some years. The anatomical structure known as the lateral aberrant thyroid has in retrospect been shown in many cases to be a very slowly growing metastatic carcinoma of the thyroid. These tumors may remain in the host for decades without ever exhibiting any neoplastic potential. Similar latent lesions of mammary glands may occur in association with carcinoma of the breast. The obvious similarity between latent carcinoma and the initiated tumor cell is apparent.

The experimental evidence for the existence of dormancy in tumor cells was shown by Fisher and Fisher in an experiment involving more than 100 rats, in which the rats were inoculated with 50 cells of a highly malignant neoplasm. If the animals were left alone for 20 weeks. they did not demonstrate the presence of the malignant cells. If a surgical laparotomy was performed, this procedure along was sufficient to bring out the malignant growth in all the operated animals, even after the inoculated cells had remained dormant in the animal for 3 months.

References

J. Berenblum and P. Shubik. The role of croton oil applications associated with a single painting of a carcinogen in tumour induction of the mouse's skin. *Brit. J. Cancer 1* (1947): 379.

N. Bloch-Shtacher, Z. Rabinowitz, and L. Sachs. Chromosomal mechanism for the induction of reversion in transformed cells. *Int. J. Cancer 9* (1972): 632.

R. K. Boutwell. Some biological aspects of skin carcinogenesis. *Progr. Exp. Tumor Res. 4* (1964): 207.

A. C. Braun. On the origin of the cancer cell. *Am. Sci. 58* (1970): 307.

A. C. Braun, and H. N. Wood. Suppression of the neoplastic state with the acquisition of specialized functions in cells, tissues and organs of crown gall teratomas of tobacco. *Proc. Natl. Acad. Sci. USA 73* (1976): 496.

B. Fisher, and E. R. Fisher. Experimental evidence in support of the dormant tumor cell. *Science 130* (1959): 918.

L. Foulds. Tumor progression and neoplastic development. In *Cellular Control Mechanisms and Cancer* (O. Mühlbock and P. Emmelot, eds.). Elsevier, Amsterdam, 1964, p. 242.

D. Gaudin, R. S. Gregg, and K. L. Yielding. DNA repair inhibition: A possible mechanism of site of cocarcinogens. *Biochem. Biophys. Res. Commun. 45* (1971): 630.

D. M. Goldenberg, R. A. Pavia, and M. C. Tsao. In vivo hybridization of human tumor and normal hamster cells. *Nature 250* (1974): 649.

I. Granberg. Chromosomes in preinvasive, microinvasive and invasive cervical carcinoma. *Hereditas 68* (1971): 165.

R. M. Hicks, J. St.J. Wakefield, and J. Chowaniec. Cocarcinogenic action of saccharin in the chemical induction of bladder cancer. *Nature 243* (1973): 347.

D. Hoffman and E. L. Wynder. A study of tobacco carcinogenesis. XI. Tumor initiators, tumor accelerators and tumor promoting activity of condensate fractions. *Cancer 27* (1971): 848.

H. M. Jensen, J. R. Rice, and S. R. Wellings. Preneoplastic lesions in the human breast. *Science 191* (1976): 295.

J. Mark. Rous sarcomas in mice: The chromosomal progression in primary tumors. *Eur. J. Cancer 5* (1969): 307.

S. Nandi, and C. M. McGrath. Mammary neoplasia in mice. *Adv. Cancer Res. 17* (1973): 353.

C. Peraino, R. J. M. Fry, E. Staffeldt, and W. E. Kisieleski. Effect of varying the exposure to phenobarbital on its enhancement of 2-acetylamino-fluorene-induced hepatic tumorigenesis in the rat. *Cancer Res. 33* (1973): 2701.

F. J. C. Roe, R. L. Carter, B. C. V. Mitchley, R. Peto, and E. Hecker. On the persistence of tumour initiation and the acceleration of tumor progression in mouse skin tumorigenesis. *Int. J. Cancer 9* (1972): 264.

M. H. Salaman. Co-carcinogenesis. *Brit. Med. Bull. 20* (1964): 139.

C. A. Waldron and W. G. Shafer. Leukoplakia revisited—a clinicopathologic study of 3,256 oral leukoplakias. *Cancer 36* (1975): 1386.

7

Host Effects
During Carcinogenesis

Endogenous Modifiers

The principal modifiers of carcinogenesis within a multicellular organism are
the hormones endogenous to the organism itself. We have previously mentioned the role of hormones and initiators, but we have not specifically
considered the possible role of these molecules during the process of carcinogenesis, either as promoting agents or as potential inhibitors. Numerous
studies have indicated the great importance of the hormonal status of the
host during the process of carcinogenesis. Some of the earliest studies on the
effect of alterations in the endocrine status of rats on their susceptibility to
hepatocarcinogens was carried out by Bielschowsky and his associates. Some
of their data are graphically presented in Figure 16. Hypophysectomy almost
completely suppresses chemical carcinogenesis in certain organs. For example,
with every chemical that has been tried except for dimethylnitrosamine,
hepatocarcinogenesis was prevented by hypophysectomy of the animal
prior to the initiation of carcinogenesis. On the other hand, under certain
conditions, administration of high levels of pituitary hormones, especially
growth hormone, dramatically increased the incidence of hepatomas in
animals fed 2-AAF. In all likelihood the reasons for these differences are
the changes in the metabolism of the carcinogens brought about by alteration in microsomal oxygenases, including those enzymes that metabolize
the procarcinogen to its active form. Studies by the Millers and their associates demonstrated that hypophysectomy decreased the urinary excretion of N-hydroxy-AAF. The excretion of this metabolite and thus presumably the conversion of AAF to its N-hydroxy derivative were largely
restored by the administration of ACTH.

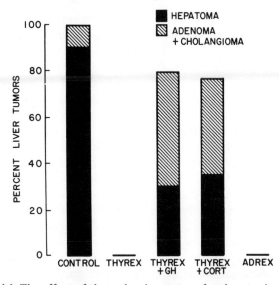

Figure 16. The effect of the endocrine status of male rats given acetylamino-fluorene on the induction of liver neoplasms. THYREX, thyroidectomized; ADREX, adrenalectomized; GH, growth hormone; CORT, cortisone. (After Bielschowsky.)

In addition to the inhibitory effect of the removal of the pituitary on hepatocarcinogenesis, thyroidectomy and adrenalectomy both completely abolished hepatocarcinogenesis induced by 2-AAF or azo dyes. Treatment of the thyroidectomized animal with numerous hormones, both steroids and polypeptides, did not relieve the inhibition. The administration of deoxy-corticosterone during azo dye carcinogenesis of adrenalectomized animals did not restore the hepatocarcinogenic effect of these dyes. However, treat-ment of thyroidectomized rats with thyroid powder did restore the carcino-genic effect of 2-AAF.

The sex of the host is also an important factor in the genesis of many types of neoplasms, both in humans and in the experimental animal. We have already discussed the generally higher incidence of neoplasms in the human male. While in both experimental animals and in humans, leukemogenesis is more frequent in the male, the most impressive experimental evidence for an effect of sex on chemical carcinogenesis is seen in the liver. Both with certain azo dyes and with 2-AAF, tumor incidence is much higher in the male animal, although N-hydroxy AAF is equally carcinogenic for both sexes in some strains of rats. In several instances, including studies with urethan and an azo dye, orchidectomy decreased the incidence of hepatic neoplasms, whereas ovariectomy increased the incidence of hepatomas. In mammary carcinogenesis, which is markedly affected by the hormonal status of the host, administration of DES stimulated a marked tumor incidence in male mice having the mammary tumor virus but did not induce many mammary neoplasms in a strain of male animals that was free of the virus.

Another factor that modifies carcinogenesis in the host is the general process of aging. As mentioned earlier, neoplasia is primarily a disease of age. Unfortunately, this fact tells us little about the actual effect of age on the induction of neoplasms by specific agents. In our previous discussion of the irreversibility of the process of initiation in mouse skin, mention was made that some evidence suggested that this process was actually reversible. However, recent studies by Van Duuren and his associates have indicated that initiation is not reversible but that the effects seen are the result of aging of the animal between the application of the carcinogen and treatment with the promoting agent some year or so later. On the other hand, some studies have indicated that aging increases the susceptibility of mouse skin to DMBA, and injection of 3-methylcholanthrene subcutaneously results in a higher incidence of tumors at the injection site in old mice than in weanling animals. Nitrosamines and azo dyes were more effective in young than in older animals in inducing hepatocellular carcinomas.

Exogenous Modifiers

We have already discussed a number of materials, termed cocarcinogens or promoting agents, during our discussion of the two-stage concept of carcinogenesis. However, other interesting effects and modifications of chemical carcinogenesis by exogenously added compounds and even by other carcinogens should be considered. We have already seen that phenobarbital enhances liver carcinogenesis by subcarcinogenic doses of 2-AAF. This drug also enhances hepatocarcinogenesis by DAB and diethylnitrosamine when administered in a manner similar to that described by Peraino. However, phenobarbital given with the carcinogen results in an inhibition of carcinogenesis. Similar effects are seen with other compounds that alter the metabolism of chemical carcinogens by the organ involved, predominantly liver, e.g., the inhibition of dimethylnitrosamine and azo dye carcinogenesis after administration of 3-methylcholanthrene. These effects are apparently due to an induction of enzymes that metabolize these carcinogens to noncarcinogenic compounds. Numerous other chemicals have been described that exhibit similar effects both on hepatocarcinogenesis and epidermal carcinogenesis. Recent studies have also demonstrated that inhibitors of RNA synthesis, such as actinomycin D, inhibit epidermal carcinogenesis in the mouse. An obvious explanation of this phenomenon, which has not yet been proven, is that initiation requires genetic transcription.

The other main source of exogenous modifiers is seen in the dietary modification of carcinogenesis in both humans and animals. The most prominent dietary modification of carcinogenesis is that of caloric restriction. This relatively simple maneuver significantly decreases tumor incidence, both experimentally induced by chemicals and spontaneously induced in animals and possibly in humans. An example is the fact that caloric restriction reduces the incidence of skin tumor induction by dibenzanthracene by more than half. In addition, caloric restriction markedly reduces the incidence of spontaneous mammary tumors as well as pulmonary neoplasms and leukemia in mice. Even when caloric restriction is initiated subsequent to the development of carcinogenesis, significant decreases in tumor incidences may result. In the human the best evidence for an effect of caloric restriction on the incidence of cancer is seen in statistics, which demonstrate that those individuals who are 25% or more over their normal weight exhibit a cancer incidence that is more than one-third higher than that of individuals who maintain their normal weight.

Studies with rats have also demonstrated that the incidence of certain spontaneous neoplasms is very much dependent on the level of protein in the diet. Marginal protein undernutrition tended to predispose animals to an early occurrence of neoplasms of the lymphoid system and high morbidity. On the other hand, protein overnutrition increased the frequency of bladder papillomas.

The effects of specific dietary constituents have also been studied in a number of experimental situations. Diethylnitrosamine carcinogenesis in the liver of the rat is enhanced by feeding a diet high in fat and deficient in certain nutritional elements that contribute methyl groups to the organism, such as choline. A similar effect is seen in hepatocarcinogenesis induced by aflatoxin B_1 and in colon cancer induced by dimethylhydrazine. A high carbohydrate diet reduces the metabolism of dimethylnitrosamine by the liver but does not affect the incidence of renal tumors induced by a single dose of this carcinogen. The early studies of the Millers and Rusch demonstrated the importance of the type of fatty acids in the diet on the incidence of azo dye-induced liver neoplasms. When animals were fed unsaturated fat together with the carcinogen, the tumor incidence was much greater than when animals were fed an isocaloric amount of saturated lipids. An interesting effect of a single amino acid is shown by the enhancement by high levels of tryptophan of hepatocarcinogenesis by diethylnitrosamine and of bladder cancer in rats fed 2-AAF. In this latter instance the difference was striking, in that very few bladder tumors were observed in animals whose diets were not supplemented with tryptophan.

The effects of vitamin deficiencies and excesses on carcinogenesis have been studied in two specific instances. Studies by the Millers and Rusch demonstrated that the riboflavin content of the diet in rats undergoing hepatocarcinogenesis by azo dyes markedly influenced the incidence of hepatomas in these animals. These investigators demonstrated that the feeding of azo dyes caused a rapid depression in the riboflavin content of the liver. Conversely, a diet high in riboflavin (10mg/kg) greatly inhibited hepatic tumor induction by DAB. Furthermore, a riboflavin analog fed together with subcarcinogenic doses of DAB resulted in significant numbers of hepatic neoplasms.

Recently a striking effect of vitamin A on epidermal and pulmonary neoplasia has been demonstrated. In the hamster given carcinogenic hydrocarbons intranasally (a regimen that induces squamous cell carcinoma of the lung), carcinogenesis can be completely inhibited by the administration of high levels of vitamin A. The feeding of a diet containing high levels of vitamin A inhibits skin carcinogenesis by dimethylbenzanthracene in mice. In addition, when vitamin A is applied directly to the skin after carcinogenesis is well under way, the morphologic type of neoplasm produced is altered, apparently as a result of the administration of the vitamin. Interestingly enough, this latter effect is inhibited by actinomycin D.

One of the most recent demonstrations of an effect of vitamin A on carcinogenesis in the rat is the inhibition of bladder carcinogenesis by N-methyl-N-nitrosourea with the synthetic retinoid, 13-cis-retinoic acid. In this example administration of the retinoic acid derivative is effective in inhibiting the incidence and extent of bladder cancer in these animals even when its administration is initiated after cessation of carcinogen dosing.

Although a major mechanism of dietary effects on hepatocarcinogenesis is probably related to the environmental control of the metabolism of carcinogens, the effect of vitamin A on skin carcinogenesis, that of tryptophan on liver and possibly bladder carcinogenesis, and most recently the effect of excess dietary copper in inhibiting renal carcinogenesis by dimethylnitrosamine are not fully understood. On the other hand, diet and nutrition may be viewed quite appropriately as modifiers or even promoting agents rather than initiators of carcinogenesis. As can be seen (vide supra), dietary components may have quite varied effects on the production of neoplasms in the host. In addition to the endogenous hormonal modification of carcinogenesis, exogenous factors may directly or indirectly affect (1) intestinal bacteria and substrates for bacterial metabolism, (2) microsomal mixed-function oxidase systems, (3) the endocrine system, (4) the immune system, (5) the availability of substrates and metabolites for cell function and proliferation, and (6) the rate of carcinogen "activation" and thereby the duration of exposure to the carcinogen. While the importance of and implications for a modifying role of nutritional and hormonal factors in human carcinogenesis are very great, much more investigation is needed in order to elucidate the many interactions between exogenous and endogenous host factors in the process of carcinogenesis in vivo.

References

E. N. Alcantara, and E. W. Speckmann. Diet, nutrition, and cancer. *Am. J. Clin. Nutr. 29* (1976): 1035.

A. S. Amulay, and R. W. O'Gara. Enhancing the effect of riboflavin analog on azo-dye carcinogenesis in rats. *J. Natl. Cancer Inst. 40* (1968): 731.

R. R. Bates, J. S. Wortham, W. B Counts, C. W. Dingman, and H. V. Gelboin. Inhibition by actinomycin D on DNA synthesis and skin tumorigenesis induced by 7,12-dimethylbenz[a]anthracene. *Cancer Res. 28* (1968): 27.

F. Bielschowsky. Neoplasia and internal environment. *Brit. J. Cancer 9* (1955): 80.

W. Bollag. Prophylaxis of chemically induced benign and malignant epithelial tumors by vitamin A acid "retinoic acid." *Eur. J. Cancer 8* (1972): 689.

W. W. Carlton, and P. S. Price. Dietary copper and the induction of neoplasms in the rat by acetylaminofluorene and dimethylnitrosamine. *Fd. Cosmet. Toxicol. 11* (1973): 827.

F. Decloitre, J. Chauveau, and M. Martin. Influence of age and 3-methylcholanthrene on azo-dye carcinogenesis and metabolism of p-dimethylaminoazobenzene in rat liver. *Int. J. Cancer 11* (1973): 676.

W. F. Dunning, M. R. Curtis, and M. E. Maun. The effect of added dietary tryptophan on the occurrence of 2-acetylaminofluorene-induced liver and bladder cancer in rats. *Cancer Res. 10* (1950): 454.

P. Ebbesen. Aging increases susceptibility of mouse skin to DMBA carcino-
    genesis independent of general immune status. *Science 183* (1974):
    217.

W. J. Eversole. Inhibition of azo dye carcinogenesis by adrenalectomy and
    treatment with deoxycorticosterone trimethylacetate. *Proc. Soc. Exp.
    Biol. Med. 96* (1957): 643.

L. M. Franks, and A. W. Carbonell. Effect of age on tumor induction in
    C57BL mice. *J. Natl. Cancer Inst. 52* (1974): 565.

G. H. Gass, J. Brown, and A. B. Okey. Carcinogenic effects of oral diethyl-
    stilbestrol on C3H male mice with and without the mammary tumor
    virus. *J. Natl. Cancer Inst. 53* (1974): 1369.

T. Kawachi, Y. Hirata, and T. Sugimura. Enhancement of N-nitrosodiethyl-
    amine hepatocarcinogenesis by L-tryptophan in rats. *Gann 59* (1968):
    523.

P. D. Lotlikar, M. Enomoto, E. C. Miller, and J. A. Miller. The effects of
    adrenalectomy, hypophysectomy and castration on the urinary meta-
    bolites of 2-acetylaminofluorene in the rat. *Cancer Res. 24* (1964):
    1835.

E. C. Miller, J. A. Miller, B. E. Kline, and H. P. Rusch. Correlation of the
    level of hepatic riboflavin with the appearance of liver tumors in rats
    fed aminoazo dyes. *J. Exp. Med. 88* (1948): 89.

J. A. Miller, B. E. Kline, H. P. Rusch, and C. A. Baumann. The carcinogen-
    icity of p-dimethylaminoazobenzene in diets containing hydrogenated
    coconut oil. *Cancer Res. 4* (1944): 153.

L. Prutkin. Modification of the effects of vitamin A acid on the skin tumor
    keratoacanthoma by applications of actinomycin D. *Cancer Res. 31*
    (1971): 1080.

M. D. Reuber. The thyroid gland and N-2-fluorenyldiacetamide carcino-
    genesis and cirrhosis of the liver in Wistar male rats. *J. Natl. Cancer
    Inst. 35* (1965): 959.

M. D. Reuber and C. W. Lee. Effect of age and sex on hepatic lesions in
    Buffalo strain rats ingesting diethylnitrosamine. *J. Natl. Cancer Inst.
    41* (1968): 1133.

A. E. Rogers and P. M. Newberne. Dietary effects on chemical carcinogenesis
    in animal models for colon and liver tumors. *Cancer Res. 35* (1975):
    3427.

A. E. Rogers, O. Sanchez, F. M. Feinsod, and P. M. Newberne. Dietary en-
    hancement of nitrosamine carcinogenesis. *Cancer Res. 34* (1974): 96.

M. H. Ross and G. Bras. Influence of protein under- and overnutrition on
    spontaneous tumor prevalence in the rat. *J. Nutr. 103* (1973): 944.

M. B. Sporn, R. A. Squire, C. C. Brown, J. M. Smith, M. L. Wenk, and S. Springer. 13-*cis*-Retinoic acid: Inhibition of bladder carcinogenesis in the rat. *Science 195* (1977): 487.

P. F. Swann and A. E. M. McLean. Cell injury and carcinogenesis. The effect of a protein-free high-carbohydrate diet on the metabolism of dimethyl-nitrosamine in the rat. *Biochem. J. 124* (1971): 283.

K. Takamiya, S-H. Chen, and H. Kitagawa. Effect of phenobarbital and DL-ethionine on 4-dimethylaminoazobenzene-metabolizing enzymes and carcinogenesis. *Gann 64* (1973): 363.

A. Tannenbaum. Effects of varying caloric intake upon tumor incidence and tumor growth. *Ann. N. Y. Acad. Sci. 49* (1954): 5.

Y. C. Toh. Physiological and biochemical reviews of sex differences and carcinogenesis with particular reference to the liver. *Adv. Cancer Res. 18* (1973): 155.

B. L. Van Duuren and S. Melchionne. Inhibition of tumorigenesis. *Progr. Exp. Tumor Res. 12* (1969): 55.

B. L. Van Duuren, A. Sivak, C. Katz, I. Seidman, and S. Melchionne. The effect of aging and interval between primary and secondary treatment in two-stage carcinogenesis in mouse skin. *Cancer Res. 35* (1975): 502.

N. Venkatesan, M. F. Argus, and J. C. Arcos. Mechanism of 3-methylchol-anthrene-induced inhibition of dimethylnitrosamine demethylase in rat liver. *Cancer Res. 30* (1970): 2556.

S. D. Vesselinovitch and N. Mihailovich. The effect of gonadectomy on the development of hepatomas induced by urethan. *Cancer Res. 27* (1967): 1788.

J. H. Weisburger, S. R. Pai, and R. S. Yamamoto. Pituitary hormones and liver carcinogenesis with N-hydroxy-N-2-fluorenylacetamide. *J. Natl. Cancer Inst. 32* (1964): 881.

8

The Natural
History of Cancer In Vivo

Cellular Replication and the Cell Cycle

As we have seen earlier (Chapter 2), the operational component of the definition of neoplasia is growth. While we have already seen that such growth may
not necessarily mean only cellular replication, it is clear that in the majority
of instances neoplastic cellular populations that we study result from the replication of one or more initiated neoplastic cells. Furthermore, the principal
component of our definition of neoplasia, that of relative autonomy, cannot
be completely divorced from the operational component of the definition.
It is quite clear that in many neoplasms, especially those of a high degree of
malignancy and anaplasia, one may point to abnormal or missing regulation
of cellular replication as the principal molecular abnormality of the neoplastic population which results in lethality to the host.

The events that occur during cellular division have for the past 125
years been a subject of fascination and intense study for the interested student and the professional biological scientist. *Mitosis,* the process of the
division of the cytoplasm and the nucleus of a cell, and *meiosis,* the process
of cellular division leading to a 50% reduction in the number of chromosomes, have been studied morphologically and, recently, biochemically in an
attempt to dissect the functional components leading up to and following this
visible sign of cellular replication. From such investigations it has become apparent that most cells undergo a series of processes that have been termed the
cell cycle and that culminate in mitosis. As can be seen in Figure 17, the cell
cycle is divided into at least four separate components, with a fifth phase, G_0,
consisting of cells that appear to leave the normal cell cycle but by specific

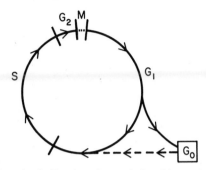

Figure 17. The cell cycle, indicating the periods of interphase (G_1), DNA synthesis (S), the period between the end of DNA synthesis and the beginning of mitosis (G_2), and the mitotic interval (M). The G_0 state is also depicted as a side extension of interphase, with the possibility that the G_0 cell may re-enter the cycle (dashed line).

stimuli can be induced to re-enter the cycle. The tendency for liver cells to divide following partial hepatectomy may be an example of the stimulation of cells in G_0 to re-enter the cycle. In addition, some cells, especially certain nerve cells of the brain, may leave the cycle and never re-enter it under any known circumstances. On the other hand, neoplastic cells may maintain a normal cycle or enter G_0, thus leaving the cycle (possibly because of major chromosomal abnormalities), never to re-enter but rather ultimately to die.

Our knowledge of the events of the cell cycle has unfortunately not led to a complete elucidation of the regulation of cellular replication in higher organisms. A number of studies, however, have indicated that certain key processes must occur during the latter phase of G_1 that signal the cell to enter the phase of DNA synthesis, the S phase. Although the endogenous and organismal regulation of cellular division is one of the principal processes of biology about which we know relatively little, it has been possible to regulate the cell cycle exogenously by various drugs and chemicals. A number of these compounds are used in the therapy of human cancer, acting most successfully on those neoplasms that have the largest number of cells entering the S phase of the cell cycle.

In the natural history of neoplastic development, cellular replication plays a major role. We have already seen its importance in the progression of neoplasia, and in this chapter we will extend the natural history of the replicating neoplastic cell population to its ultimate conclusion, the metastatic neoplastic cell.

The Clonality of Neoplasms

The growth characteristics of neoplasms in vivo have never been adequately investigated. Most studies rely on a simple external measurement from radiologic studies to determine the volume of a neoplasm and any changes therein as a function of time. On the basis of such investigations, the doubling time of the average human neoplasm has been reported to be between 50 and 60 days. For squamous cell neoplasms and adenocarcinomas this figure was reported as 82 and 166 days, respectively. However, such figures are relatively meaningless unless one can determine other characteristics of neoplastic growth. One of the more significant of such characteristics is the question of the clonality of a neoplasm.

According to Fialkow, one might expect that a neoplasm arising as a consequence of one or a few relatively rare random events would have a clonal or single cell origin. Multiclonal or multicellular origins of neoplasms would be expected if the neoplastic transformation of many cells occurred relatively simultaneously, such as one might see with an infectious agent, e.g., a virus. Since the virus etiology of human neoplasia has been established only in the case of two neoplasms, by this reasoning most human cancers should be monoclonal. As seen in Table 10, this is the case.

The determination of the clonality of a neoplasm results from a study of specific aspects of its biochemistry or its karyotype. In chronic myelogenous leukemia, in which the leukemic cells all possess the Philadelphia chromosome, a monoclonal origin would be expected. Myelomas are almost always found to produce only a single type of immunoglobulin; based on our knowledge of immunobiology, myelomas presumably arise from a single or very few cells. However, the best evidence in support of the monoclonal derivation of those neoplasms seen in Table 11 (Chapter 10) depends on the investigations of the isozymic forms of sex chromosome X-linked marker enzymes in the cells. As can be seen from Figure 18, in the normal mammalian female early during embryonic development but following meiosis, one of the two X chromosomes in each cell is repressed. The mechanism of this repression is unknown, but it culminates, in the fully developed organism, in a mosaic cellular pattern consisting of a number of populations of cells expressing the genes on one X chromosome while the remaining cellular populations of the organism express the genes on the other X chromosome. If an individual is heterozygous (different alleles or copies of the gene in each of the two chromosomes), then some cells will express one form of the gene and other cells the other. In relation to the monoclonal derivation of neoplasms, some females are mosaic for two isozymic forms of the enzyme,

Table 10. Single or Multiple Cell Origin of Tumors Determined with G-6-PD Markers[a]

Single cell origin proved or very probable		Multicellular origin	
Neoplasm	No. studied	Neoplasm	No. studied
Benign		Hereditary	
Uterine leiomyoma	184	Neurofibroma	14
Common wart	6	Trichoepithelioma	12
Thyroid adenoma	4	Carcinoma (non-hereditary)	
Lipoma	3	Colon	1
Salivary gland adenoma	2	Cervix, invasive(?)	2
Ovarian teratoma	3	Lymphoma	
Chronic myelocytic leukemia	5	Burkitt	1
Lymphoma			
Burkitt	42		
Reticulum cell sarcoma	2		
Lymphosarcoma	1		
Plasma cell neoplasia	3		
Paroxysmal nocturnal hemoglobinuria	2		
Carcinoma			
Bladder	1		
Nasopharynx	2		
Thyroid	5		
Palate	3		
Cervix			
Noninvasive	7		
Invasive	8		
Bowen's disease of vulva	1		
Melanoma	2		
Neuroblastoma	1		
Nephroblastoma	1		
Bilateral medullary carcinoma of thyroid	1		

[a]After Fialkow (1974).

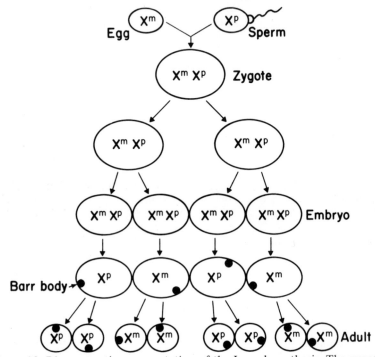

Figure 18. Diagrammatic representation of the Lyon hypothesis. The zygote (fertilized egg) is depicted as that of a female inheriting one X chromosome from the mother (X^m) and the other from the father (X^p). These chromosomes are inherited in daughter cells, but at some early time in embryogenesis there occurs a difference in behavior of each of the two X chromosomes in each somatic cell such that only one X chromosome remains active in each cell and its subsequent daughters. The other X chromosome is inactive and becomes the Barr body as noted in the figure. Thus the adult female becomes a mosaic with a number of cells expressing the genes of X^p, while others express those of X^m. (After Fialkow, 1974).

glucose-6-phosphate dehydrogenase, resulting from the repression of one or the other X chromosome in individual cells during early embryonic life as stated by the Lyon hypothesis. Thus, if a neoplasm arising in such a mosaic individual contains only a single form of this enzyme, it is likely to have resulted from a clonal initiation.

On the other hand, it is difficult to rule out the possibility that the early neoplastic transformation occurred in many cells but that then one or very few cells attained a growth advantage and overgrew the vast majority of the population. In any event, the clonal history of neoplasms is an important problem, the elucidation of which will be helpful in our understanding of the natural history of the disease.

Prognostication of the Natural History of Neoplasms

Primarily for diagnostic reasons, malignant neoplasms in the human have been divided according to histologic *grade*. The grading of neoplasms by the pathologist can be done most easily with certain types of carcinomas, especially epidermoid carcinomas. A grade-1 carcinoma is a highly differentiated, slightly anaplastic carcinoma. At the other extreme, a grade-4 carcinoma is histologically very similar to a carcinosarcoma, a highly malignant, aneuploid, rapidly growing neoplasm. Grades 2 and 3 are intermediate stages, and their designation is obviously somewhat subjective. The histologic grading of the tumor is always done by grading the most anaplastic histologic areas of the neoplasm.

The staging of neoplasms has been employed to characterize the invasive and extensive characteristics of neoplasms. For example, in the case of carcinoma of the cervix, a stage-zero tumor would be a carcinoma in situ. Carcinoma in situ, of course, would not have invaded deeply into the cervix, although it might have invaded into the surrounding epithelium. Such intraepithelial invasion may also be seen in Paget's disease of the nipple, which heralds a malignant neoplasm of the breast. Stages I–III of invasive cervical carcinoma depend on whether the tumor is confined to the uterus (1), extends into neighboring regions such as the vagina and uterine ligaments (2), or shows distant metastases (3). In determining the results of surgical and radiological treatment, the determination of the effects based on the initial stage of the neoplasm can give the physician a much clearer picture of how efficacious the therapy is.

The mechanisms of invasive neoplastic growth are not entirely clear as yet. Earlier studies suggested that the motility and rapidity of growth of the neoplastic cell, together with a probable capacity for proteolysis and a decrease in pH brought about by high glycolysis of the tumor, were responsible for its ability to invade normal tissue. Recently the phenomenon of contact inhibition of movement, wherein normal cells are "inhibited" in growth and motion by one another, has been described both in vivo and in vitro. Studies on neoplastic cells in culture have shown that tumor cells in most instances have lost the capacity to be contact inhibited.

With regard to contact inhibition of cells, it is important to define what is being inhibited and what is being contacted in what environment. Originally, the term referred to effects on cell-to-cell contact and locomotion. More recently, the term has also involved cell overlap during growth as well as colony expansion and the "contact inhibition of cell division." The lack of contact inhibition of cell division and the "piling up" of cells have been used as criteria to score cells as transformed in vitro. The mechanism of contact inhibition is not clear, although it undoubtedly involves surface membrane factors and structures that differ between normal and neoplastic cells. Some of these factors involve the capacity of cells to interact with certain plant lectins in vitro, although there is no clear correlation between cell agglutination by such lectins and the cells' capacity to be contact-inhibited.

Metastases: Incidence and Mechanism

As noted earlier, a metastatic tumor is one that originates from and is physically separated from the primary neoplastic growth. The capacity of malignant tumors to metastasize is perhaps the major feature of their lethality to the host.

Routes of Metastases

Anatomically, a number of pathways for metastatic cells are possible. The most obvious is the blood circulation, in which tumor cells gain entrance to the vascular system and then are carried by the bloodstream to new sites where they initiate growth. Usually this new growth begins in small capillaries, where tumor cells are caught and begin to invade through the capillary endothelium to initiate a new growth. It is obvious from present studies that the number of cells that enter the bloodstream is far greater than the number that ever give rise to metastatic lesions. The phenomenon of "canceremia" or tumor cells in the blood has recently been studied through the use of blood filtrates, in which the number of tumor cells per milliliter may be estimated. In advanced cases of neoplasia this number is quite high, whereas in early tumor growth there may be virtually no tumor cells within the blood vascular system. From experimental studies it would appear that only when a neoplasm reaches a certain critical size does it begin to shed cells into the bloodstream. Of the cells entering the bloodstream, considerably less than 0.01% ever give rise to any metastatic lesions.

Another common route of metastatic cells is the lymphatic system, in which the flow of tumor cells, although considerably slower than in the bloodstream, is probably of a similar magnitude. Some tumors may implant in other sites by mere physical movement from one site to another. This is commonly seen in certain ovarian or gastrointestinal tumors, with resultant implantation of neoplastic cells from one side of the peritoneal cavity to the other. A similar sort of implantation is probably the mechanism responsible for the appearance of accessory spleens; i.e., intraabdominal splenic tissue separate from the spleen itself.

With the advent of numerous surgical techniques, a new type of metastasis has become known. If the surgeon is not careful, his knife may enter the neoplasm and become covered with tumor cells, which may be carried to and implanted at another site in the surgical field. It would appear that this accounts for the reappearance of tumors in the operative site some months or years after the initial surgery in the treatment of a specific neoplasm. In addition, manipulation of the tumor during surgery may initiate both vascular and lymphatic metastic lesions. However, now that these problems are apparent, most surgeons take extreme care to prevent the occurrence of such metastases during curative resections.

In experimental oncology, the analog to surgical metastasis is the tumor transplant. Clearly, in the original behavioristic classification of neoplasms, the distinguishing feature of the metastatic capability of the malignant neoplasm is reflected in its transplantability. In some instances, however, it has been possible to transplant neoplasms that have not been shown to be behavioristically malignant in the original primary host. This further points out the artificiality of the behavioristic classification to the experimental oncologist.

Incidences and Sites of Tumor Metastases

As stated previously, the number of metastatic cells that give rise to metastatic lesions is extremely small. Metastases usually appear in the adjacent lymph nodes or in the lung or liver, the site depending on where the tumor originates. Certain tumors may have a predisposition, because of their anatomical location, to metastasize to certain organs. Cancer of the lung not uncommonly metastasizes to the brain, possibly because of the invasion of tumor cells into the pulmonary veins. Metastatic cells may then enter the carotid arteries. Carcinoma of the breast or lung regularly metastasizes to the adrenal glands, and carcinoma of the prostate frequently metastasizes to bones, particularly the vertebrae. Very few metastatic lesions occur in some organs, for example, the spleen and thymus. In the case of the thymus, this

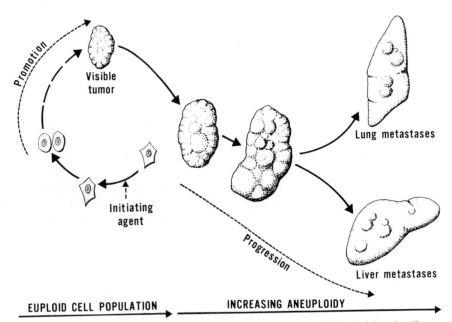

Figure 19. The natural history of neoplasia beginning with the initiated cell resulting from the application of an initiating agent (carcinogen) and subsequent promotion to a visible tumor with progression of this neoplasm to malignancy. The relationship to karyotype is presented as a generalization on the lower arrows. The reader should again be cautioned that not all neoplastic cells undergo this entire natural history. It is theoretically possible, although this has not yet been definitively shown, that some neoplasms, such as those induced in animals by radiation or high doses of chemical carcinogens, may enter this sequence in the stage of progression, exhibiting aneuploidy, and thus bypass the early euploid cell stage in the natural history of neoplasia.

is probably because of its peculiar vascular system. Since tumor cells have difficulty in establishing metastatic lesions in the spleen, the destructive capacity of spleen cells probably contributes to this difficulty and prevents most metastatic lesions.

In most experimentally produced neoplasms, the animal is sacrificed prior to the occurrence of metastatic lesions. Therefore, it is not uncommon to find an animal harboring a histologically malignant neoplasm with no evidence of metastatic lesions. Were the animal to be allowed to die of the cancer, the incidence of metastatic lesions would be much higher in such experimental situations.

Mechanisms of Metastases

The exact mechanism for the production and growth of metastatic lesions is not known (see Figure 19). In early studies it was suggested that decreased cellular cohesion, possibly resulting from decreased intercellular concentration of calcium, accounted for the ability of tumor cells to metastasize. One may also invoke the absence of contact inhibition as an explanation for the fact that tumor cells may grow and invade into adjacent tissues. However, it is now apparent that probably only certain cells of primary neoplasms have the capacity to initiate metastatic growth. In virtually every case examined, metastatic lesions exhibit aneuploid karyotypes. It would thus appear that aneuploidy gives to the neoplastic cell a definite growth advantage, which allows the cell to initiate metastatic growth. Since most, if not all, malignant neoplasms have at least some aneuploid cells in their population, it is probably these cells that ultimately give rise to surviving metastatic clones. Presumably metastatic cells having a normal karyotype are not suited for metastatic growth and thus seldom survive the rigors of clonal initiation.

A number of other factors have also been shown to be active in the formation of metastases. Among these are the number of platelets in the blood, fibrin formation, the size of the hematogenous metastatic tumor cell clumps, and the immune status of the host. Although all of these factors undoubtedly interplay with one another, their number and complexity indicate, together with the known phenomenon of canceremia, that the successful initiation of a metastatic growth is by no means a simple process.

It should be recalled that certain normal tissues also have the capacity to metastasize. The placenta uniformly metastasizes during the last several months of pregnancy, and in individuals who have died during this period, metastatic cells are found in the pulmonary vasculature. Undoubtedly, the cells die after the birth of the child because of alteration in the hormonal environment. That accessory spleens are probably metastases from normal spleens has already been discussed. In certain cases of trauma, especially after fractures of bone, fat cells may metastasize to other parts of the organism, sometimes with extremely deleterious effects.

The Metastatic Cell as the Ultimate
in the Natural History of Neoplasia

In Figure 19 is seen a diagram of the natural history of neoplasia as the student may now perceive it, beginning with the process of initiation, extending through the promotion of the initiated cell to a visible tumor, and then following the natural progression of this tumor, usually a benign neoplasm, to the ultimate expression of malignancy, that of distant metastases. At the bottom of the figure may be seen the concomitant relationship of the cellular karyotype extending throughout this process. Exactly where the progeny of the initiated cell(s) begin to exhibit chromosomal aberrations is obviously quite variable from one situation to another. Furthermore, the student should remember that, although this diagram suggests monoclonality of neoplasms, examples of multiclonal neoplasms may well follow the same natural history although in a somewhat more complicated manner.

The student should also realize that not every neoplastic cell resulting from the transformation of a normal cell must follow this entire series of steps. It is know that some agents, including chemical, radiation and biologic agents, produce aneuploid neoplastic cellular populations very early if not coincident with the transformation process. However, in the case of many human neoplasms it is likely that the natural history of such lesions is similar to that shown in Figure 19.

References

R. Baserga (ed.). *The Cell Cycle and Cancer.* Marcel Dekker, New York, 1971.
S. Baylin, D.S. Gann, and S. H. Hsu. Clonal origin of inherited medullary thyroid carcinoma and pheochromocytoma. *Science 193* (1976): 321.
H. Ben-Basset, M. Inbar, and L. Sachs. Changes in the structural organization of the surface membrane in malignant cell transformation. *J. Membrane Biol. 6* (1971): 183.
J. W. Berg, S. I. Hajdu, and F. W. Foote. The prevalence of latent cancers in cancer patients. *Arch. Pathol. 91* (1971): 183.
M. M. Burger and A. R. Goldberg. Identification of a tumor-specific determinant on neoplastic cell surfaces. *Proc. Natl. Acad. Sci. USA 57* (1967): 359.
A. Charbit, E. P. Malaise, and M. Tubiana. Relation between the pathological nature and the growth rate of human tumors. *Eur. J. Cancer 7* (1971): 307.
P. J. Fialkow. The origin and development of humor tumor studies with cell markers. *N. Eng. J. Med. 291* (1974): 26.

P. J. Fialkow, R. W. Sagebiel, S. M. Gartler, and D. L. Rimoin. Multiple cell origin of hereditary neurofibromas. *New Eng. J. Med. 284* (1971): 298.

I. J. Fidler. Immune stimulation-inhibition of experimental cancer metastasis. *Cancer Res. 34* (1974): 491.

B. Fisher and E. R. Fisher. Anticoagulants and tumor cell lodgement. *Cancer Res. 27* (1967): 421.

B. Fisher and E. R. Fisher. Experimental evidence in support of the dormant tumor cell. *Science 130* (1959): 918.

B. Fisher, E. R. Fisher, and A. Sakai. Experimental studies of factors influencing hepatic metastases. XV. Effect of neonatal thymectomy. *Cancer Res. 25* (1965): 993.

B. Fisher, E. R. Fisher, and N. Feduska. Trauma and the localization of tumor cells. *Cancer 20* (1967): 23.

G. J. Gasic, T. B. Gasic, and C. C. Stewart. Antimetastatic effects associated with platelet reduction. *Proc. Natl. Acad. Sci. USA 61* (1968): 46.

K. Laki. Fibrinogen and metastases. *J. Med. 5* (1974): 32.

L. A. Liotta, J. Kleinerman, and G. M. Saidel. The significance of hematogenous tumor cell clumps in the metastatic process. *Cancer Res. 36* (1976): 889.

E. Martz and M. S. Steinberg. Contact inhibition of what? An analytical review. *J. Cell. Physiol. 81* (1973): 25.

G. C. Mueller. Biochemical events in the animal cell cycle. *Fed. Proc. 28* (1969): 1780.

D. M. Prescott. The cell cycle and the control of cellular reproduction. *Adv. Genet. 18* (1976): 99.

9

The Pathogenesis of
Neoplastic Transformation In Vitro

Although the explantation of cells from a multicellular organism into an extraorganismal environment, i.e., tissue culture, had been known since the beginning of this century, it was not until the early 1940s that Earle and his associates attempted to induce carcinogenesis in cultured mammalian cells. These now classic experiments, which were carried out by the addition of polycyclic hydrocarbons to cultures of mouse fibroblasts, were monitored by the inoculation of treated and untreated cell cultures into host animals. Unfortunately the results of these experiments were ambiguous, since neoplasms arose in the test animals whether treated or control cultured cells were inoculated. As a result, the question of the feasibility of in vitro carcinogenesis lay dormant for almost two decades.

Techniques of Tissue Culture

It is not our objective to discuss the methodology of cell and organ culture in extenso. The interested student is referred to several of the bibliographic references. However, it is important for the student to understand the difference between organ culture and cell culture. In the former, fragments of organs or even whole organs are removed from the organism and their viability and organization maintained in an artificial environment. One of the most famous instances of organ culture was the maintenance of a chicken heart in a functionally beating condition by Alexis Carrel during the early years of this century. Alternatively, fragments of organs can be maintained for some period of time in culture with their microscopic anatomy remaining essentially identical with that seen in the organ in vivo.

On the other hand, cell culture involves the isolation and/or dispersion of cells from organs and tissues, with their subsequent cultivation as cellular populations with little regard to their original morphology and functionality. Such cell cultures may be cloned, i.e., single cells isolated and allowed to proliferate to a visible colony. Quantitative measurements and genetic studies may be performed relatively easily with cell cultures, provided the cells either are available in significant quantity or replicate quite readily in the culture environment.

The media in which organ and cell cultures are maintained or stimulated to grow are quite complex, consisting of numerous nutrients of known composition as well as, in almost all instances, numerous materials of unknown chemical composition such as serum, partial protein hydrolysates, and tissue extracts. A few types of cells have been cultivated in chemically defined media, the most recent examples being primary cultures of liver cells. The term "primary culture" indicates those cells obtained directly from the animal and cultured in the specific system under study. Secondary and transfer cultures refer to the subsequent cultivation of cells, with the inoculum taken from cells already in culture.

In general, cells within organ cultures maintain all of the genetic and functional capabilities of comparable cells existing in vivo. In cell culture, however, especially of tissues from certain types of animals such as rodents, the natural history of cells transferred and cultivated for long periods is that of karyotypic and biochemical changes, usually in the direction of increased aneuploidy and decreased biochemical differentiation. Cells from a single source that have been maintained in culture for many transfer generations and are immortal are referred to as cell lines. Such cells may be frozen at liquid air temperatures and maintained in this state for years with relatively efficient recovery of viability on thawing. A few primary cell cultures have also been successfully maintained in this way, but organ cultures do not readily survive such treatment.

Carcinogenesis in Organ Cultures

Attempts at the induction of neoplasia in organ cultures were made in a reasonably systematic way by Heidelberger and his associates in the early part of the last decade. These investigators attempted to induce carcinomas in organ cultures of rat prostate by the addition of carcinogenic polycyclic hydrocarbons to the cultures. Although significant morphologic changes occurred, including squamous metaplasia and cytologic anaplasia, no neoplasms were produced when the cultures exhibiting such changes were inoculated back into suitable mouse hosts. Similar changes have been produced by other investigators in organ cultures of rat trachea. Numerous investigators have attempted to transform fetal cells in organ cultures and then to reimplant these into suitable hosts. In some instances neoplasms arose; however, a difficulty of these experiments was the question of whether or not the original carcinogen had been completely removed from the cultures prior to their inoculation into suitable hosts. Obviously, if the latter had not occurred, one would be dealing merely with carcinogenesis in vivo.

Neoplastic "Transformation" in Cell Culture

It was almost 20 years after the pioneering studies of Earle and his associates that Berwald and Sachs demonstrated the "transformation" of hamster embryo cells growing in cell cultures. After treatment of such cultures with methylcholanthrene or benzpyrene, with subsequent cloning, cell colonies formed that exhibited morphologic characteristics different from control or solvent-treated cells. The morphologic characteristics demonstrated were those of small, fusiform cells that grew in an irregular crisscross pattern and did not appear to exhibit contact inhibition of movement or growth, as was found in untreated control cells in culture (Figure 20). However, when these investigators attempted their experiments in cultures of mouse cells, control cultures had almost as many transformants as did cells in cultures treated with carcinogenic hydrocarbons. This question of spontaneous transformation in cell culture, although known to exist since Earle's experiments, became a major problem in all studies of neoplastic transformation in cell culture, and to this day we do not completely understand the mechanism of "spontaneous transformation" in cell culture.

Some of the characteristics of the experiments by Berwald and Sachs were quite interesting, especially the fact that the incidence of transformation was extremely high, exceeding 80% in some experiments. This argued rather strongly that the mechanism of the transformation by chemicals was not simple mutation, because of the high incidence of conversion. These authors also demonstrated the in vitro transformation of hamster embryo cells by X-irradiation and by infection with oncogenic papovaviruses.

Later studies in this country by Heidelberger with the prostate system (vide supra) confirmed and extended these earlier investigations. In Heidelberger's studies the organ cultures treated with hydrocarbons were dispersed

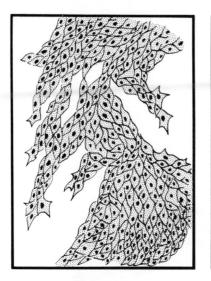

NORMAL   TRANSFORMED

Figure 20. An artist's conception of the microscopic appearance of normal and transformed cells in culture. The single cell layer of spindle cells is characteristic of the normal, which ultimately exhibits contact inhibition of replication, whereas the transformed cells exhibit cytologic anaplasia and "piling up" of one cell on another, with lack of contact inhibition of replication.

into cell suspensions, and cell lines were produced that were transformed. DiPaolo has also confirmed the work of Sachs and has demonstrated that by inhibiting the cellular toxicity of carcinogenic hydrocarbons in hamster embryo cell cultures with various noncarcinogenic chemicals, one may dissociate the transforming property from the toxic metabolic property of carcinogenic hydrocarbons.

In addition to these systems, which are concerned primarily with mesenchymal cell transformation, there have been reports of the transformation of liver cells in culture. Unfortunately, many of these studies are rather confusing, since the usual hepatocarcinogens utilized for hepatocarcinogenesis in vivo are not effective in transforming these cell cultures. Their proximate forms, as well as other carcinogens such as polycyclic hydrocarbons, alkylating agents, and the powerful carcinogen, nitroquinoline oxide, are effective in transforming cells in cultures derived from liver. In one report aflatoxin has been shown to induce the transformation of liver cells in culture. There is still significant question about whether or not such cells are truly hepatic, since in almost all reported instances the neoplasms produced on inoculation of the transformed cells in vivo were not hepatocellular carcinomas.

Criteria for Neoplastic
Transformation In Vitro

One of the significant critical points in the study of transformation in vitro is that it is obviously impossible to utilize the usual criteria of carcinogenesis in vivo to identify neoplastic cells. The morphologic changes seen initially by Berwald and Sachs were claimed to be the result of oncogenesis; however, such claims could be substantiated only if the cells could grow as neoplasms in a suitable host. Thus there has been much discussion of the criteria for neoplastic transformation in vitro. To date no universal criteria have been accepted, although most scientists in the field agree on a number of characteristics. The more important of these criteria may be listed as follows:

1. Production of biologically malignant neoplasms in vivo by inoculation of 10^6 or fewer cells into syngeneic or immunodeficient hosts, in the absence of neoplasms produced by inoculation of comparable numbers of cells not treated with the "transforming" agent. Some "transformed" cell lines do not conform to this criterion, and some embryonic cells injected into immunosuppressed or syngeneic hosts will grow to the size of a gross tumor. The time of growth of transformed cells to detectable size in the syngeneic host may vary tremendously.

2. "Immortality" of transformed cells in culture. This is characteristic of many biologically neoplastic cells, although in some instances those having "immortality" in vitro do not give rise to tumors in vivo.

3. Growth of transformed cells in soft agar. With the exception of some mouse cell strains, e.g., Heidelberger's stain C3H/10T1/2 and transformed mouse prostate cells, transformed cells exhibiting this characteristic also produce neoplasms on inoculation into a suitable host. On the other hand, a number of biologically neoplastic tissues grown in vivo will not grow in soft agar in culture.

4. Colonies of transformed cells exhibit morphologic and growth characteristics in culture different from those of normal cells grown in culture. "Nontransformed" cells grow in an "ordered" way, whereas transformed cells tend to "pile up" with crisscross patterns and a higher degree of pleomorphism. However, this criterion relates only to fibroblastic cells grown in culture. So few epithelial cells have been transformed in culture that morphological criteria of transformation for epithelial cells have not been determined accurately.

5. Loss of "contact inhibition" of cell replication under specific conditions of media and plating and increase in saturation density by transformed cells. Again, this characteristic appears not to hold for epithelial cell cultures, and a significant number of nontransformed cells in culture demonstrate no contact inhibition.

6. "Transformed" cells in many, but not all, instances may be agglutinated by plant lectins. Not all agglutinated cells, however, demonstrate biological neoplasia in vivo.

7. Cells "transformed" by chemicals or viruses in culture exhibit antigenic alterations. "Spontaneous transformants" show no antigenic alterations.

8. Transformed cells may show karyotypic changes. However, cell lines that produce no tumors in vivo may be quite aneuploid, as are many "revertants" in culture.

9. "Transformed" cells usually have a greater efficiency of cloning than nontransformed cells.

10. Production of plasminogen activator (see Chapter 10) by many, but not all, transformed cells.

It is clear that the ultimate standard of the neoplastic transformation is still the establishment of malignant neoplasms growing in vivo, but all of the characteristics listed above apply to transformed cells in vitro and, taken together, they strongly support the identification of a clone of cells transformed in vitro as biologically neoplastic. Still, no single criterion can mark a cell transformed in culture as biologically neoplastic.

Other Characteristics of Neoplastic
Transformation in Cell Culture

One of the most interesting characteristics of the neoplastic transformation in cell culture was initially described by Berwald and Sachs. They demonstrated that, unless the carcinogen remained in the culture medium for a period of time at least equivalent to that of a single cell cycle of the cells being treated, no transformation would occur. This finding led to the demonstration in cell culture of the requirement for at least one round of cell division for the neoplastic transformation to be "fixed." This same phenomenon held true for both DNA tumor virus and X-irradiation-induced transformation in cell culture. Since that time other reports have suggested that in certain circumstances transformation may be fixed without a complete round of cell division, whereas Sachs and his associates have recently suggested that at least two cell divisions are required to fix transformation by chemicals in cell culture. In at least one system, Heidelberger and his associates have suggested that transformation of a cell is most efficient when the carcinogen is applied just prior to the onset of DNA synthesis.

Although it is clear that the original two-stage hypothesis of Berenblum is not easily demonstrated in cell culture, some recent investigations in cell culture have indicated that after treatment of cells initially transformed with polycyclic hydrocarbons by phorbol esters, the efficiency of transformation and the ability of the transformed cells to grow in soft agar is significantly enhanced. It is rather difficult to extrapolate from these initial experiments, but other studies have demonstrated that transformed cells, which could be identified by morphologic changes, did not fit all of the criteria listed above. For example, some morphologically transformed cells were not immortal. As indicated above, some cells that exhibit morphologic changes and even karyotypic abnormalities do not grow as neoplastic cells in vivo. Thus we may be able in the in vitro situation to separate various essential components of the process of neoplastic transformation.

In a very recent series of experiments Mondal and Heidelberger have demonstrated that irradiation of mouse cells in culture by ultraviolet light followed by treatment with phorbol esters in vitro results in cell transformation. Since neither of these regimens alone produces cell transformation, nor does pretreatment with phorbol esters followed by ultraviolet irradiation, this system is almost completely analogous to the initiation-promotion sequence in skin. Here, ultraviolet light acts essentially as a pure initiator and the phorbol esters as a noncarcinogenic promoting agent.

One of the most interesting findings resulting from studies of the neoplastic transformation in vivo is the phenomenon of reversion (see Chapter 6).
Sachs and his associates demonstrated this very early in their investigations
and were able to show that in some instances the incidence of reversion from
the morphologically transformed state to a morphologically normal cellular
appearance (Figure 20) was exceedingly high (10-20%); this finding also
argued against the transformation process as the result of a single gene mutation but did not rule out the role of chromosomal changes in the genesis of
transformation. Such revertants occur even in virus-transformed cells, and the
reverted cells still possess viral information within their DNA. Recently Sachs
and his associates have demonstrated that most, if not all, reverted cells exhibit significant karyotypic abnormalities, usually characterized by a high
degree of polyploidy. They have proposed a model that implies that the balance of gene dosage for the expression and suppression of the neoplastic
transformation is critical in the formation of revertants. Such a concept
would certainly conform to our knowledge of karyotypes of neoplasms in
vivo and even of those neoplasms known to undergo reversion or differentiation in vivo.

Genetic Studies of Neoplasia In Vitro:
Somatic Cell Hybridization

Since one of the principal mechanisms proposed for the neoplastic transformation is that the process results from specific genetic alterations in the
cellular genome, cell culture potentially offers a system in which to study
directly the genetics of the neoplastic transformation. This potentiality was
theoretically realized when the phenomenon of somatic cell hybridization or
cell fusion was discovered. In this process (shown diagrammatically in Figure
21) two cells from the same or different species are fused, usually in the
presence of inactivated Sendai virus or certain lipids, resulting in the formation of a single cell with two nuclei termed a heterokaryon when two different cells are fused. If cells of the same type are fused, the product is termed
a homokaryon. The binucleate heterokaryon contains all of the genetic apparatus from each of the two original cells. After DNA synthesis, mitosis
occurs with a mixing of the chromosomes from each of the two nuclei and
subsequent formation of a single nucleus containing most or all of the chromosomes from the two donor cells. As this heterokaryon continues to undergo successive cell divisions, generally chromosomes of one or the other of the

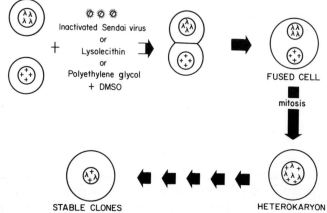

Figure 21. Outline of the fusion of somatic cells in the laboratory. The chromosomes of each of the two cells arising from two different species are denoted by + and λ. After fusion of the cells and subsequent mitosis, the heterokaryon is seen to contain the chromosomes of both cells but after subsequent replication stable clones with a reduced number of chromosomes occur.

donor cell nuclei are lost until a stable heterokaryon is obtained, usually consisting of virtually all of the chromosomes of one donor cell and one or only a few chromosomes from the other. By suitable chromosome identification one can determine the origin of each of the chromosomes of the heterokaryon.

Harris and his associates were among the first to utilize this technique in an attempt to determine whether or not the inheritance of the malignant state in such heterokaryons acted as a dominant or recessive trait. In their studies of the fusion between malignant and nonmalignant cells, malignancy behaved as a recessive character although fusion of a variety of malignant cells failed to demonstrate any complementation of the supposed genetic trait since all such resulting heterokaryons were malignant. If fusion of normal cells with virally transformed cells occurred, the resulting heterokaryon was neoplastic if it possessed integrated viral information within its genome. The studies of Harris and his associates have been questioned by other investigators whose results suggest that malignancy may be a dominant trait in that hybrids between malignant and normal cells all were shown to produce neoplasms in suitable hosts. More recent investigations by Stanbridge have upheld the original thesis of Harris and his associates, using normal and malignant human cells for the production of homokaryons. The studies of Harris also showed that if a normal-malignant hybrid lost many of its chromosomes, the neoplastic state would reappear; this indicates that the normal cells may contain specific suppressors of malignancy. Sachs and his associates have suggested similar mechanisms, even relating the suppressor function to specific chromo-somes within hamster cells (vide supra). While these hypotheses are very pro-vocative and possess significant implications as to the nature and ultimate control of the neoplastic transformation, the available data are insufficient at the present time to substantiate any general conclusions on the basis of the experimental information available.

References

Y. Berwald and L. Sachs. In vitro cell transformation with chemical carcino-gens. *Nature 200* (1963): 1182.

C. M. Croce, D. Aden, and H. Koprowski. Tumorigenicity of mouse-human diploid hybrids in nude mice. *Science 190* (1975): 1200.

J. A. DiPaolo, P. J. Donovan, and R. L. Nelson. Transformation of hamster cells in vitro by polycyclic hydrocarbons without cytotoxicity. *Proc. Natl. Acad. Sci. USA 68* (1971): 2958.

A. E. Freeman and R. J. Huebner. Problems in interpretation of experimental evidence of cell transformation. *J. Natl. Cancer Inst. 50* (1973): 303.

H. Harris. Cell fusion and the analysis of malignancy. *J. Natl. Cancer Inst. 48* (1972): 851.

C. Heidelberger. Chemical oncogenesis in culture. *Adv. Cancer Res. 18* (1973): 317.

H. Katsuta and T. Takaoka. Parameters for malignant transformation of mam-malian cells treated with chemical carcinogens in tissue culture. In *Topics in Chemical Carcinogenesis* (W. Nakahara, S. Takayama, T. Sugimura, and S. Odashima, eds.). University of Tokyo Press, Tokyo, 1973, p. 389.

P. F. Kruse, Jr. and M. K. Patterson, Jr. (eds.). *Tissue Culture – Methods and Applications.* Academic, New York, 1973.

C. Lasne, A. Gentil, and I. Chouroulinkov. Two-state malignant transforma-

S. Mondal and C. Heidelberger. Transformation of C3H/10T½ Mouse embryo fibroblasts by UV irradiation and a phorbol ester. *Nature 260* (1976): 710.

H. C. Pitot. Criteria of neoplastic transformation. In *Carcinogenesis Testing of Chemicals.* CRC Press, Inc., Cleveland, 1974, p. 113.

L. Sachs. Regulation of membrane changes, differentiation, and malignancy in carcinogenesis. *Harvey Lectures 68* (1974): 1.

E. J. Stanbridge. Suppression of malignancy in human cells. *Nature 260* (1976): 17.

F. Wiener, G. Klein, and H. Harris. The analysis of malignancy by cell fusion. VI. Hybrids between different tumor cells. *J. Cell. Sci. 16* (1974): 189.

10

The Biochemistry of Cancer

The Biochemistry of Neoplasia In Vivo

Although the discoveries of chemical, physical, and biological carcinogenic agents have been perhaps the most exciting and significant in our understanding of the causation of cancer and of many aspects of its prevention, nothing has intrigued the biological scientist more than the biochemistry of the cancer cell in relation to that of normal cells. The first hint of this interest by biochemists in the cancer problem was shown during the first two decades of this century when the structures of nucleotides and sugar phosphates were just becoming known to the biochemical scientists. In a recent review Potter has detailed much of the historical development of biochemical investigations in the cancer problem (Table 11). Just as the initial morphologic and biological studies of neoplasia during the latter half of the last century resulted in three principal theoretical explanations of the neoplastic process (see Chapter 1), the development of biochemistry has given rise to a series of hypotheses on the biochemical nature of neoplasia as well as the biochemical mechanisms that result in the conversion of a normal to a neoplastic cell. In the first part of this chapter we will consider several of the more well-known biochemical theories of the nature and genesis of neoplasia. However, the reader will notice that the basic biochemical lesion(s) essential to the neoplastic transformation have eluded biochemists and molecular biologists up to this time.

Table 11. Historical Perspectives in Cancer Biochemistry[a]

Period	Cancer Biochemistry	General Biochemistry
1913-23	Enzyme differences	1918, 3' RN-tides from RNA 1918, Fructose 6-P 1922, Glucose 6-P
1923-33	Aerobic glycolysis-respiratory defect (Warburg theory)	1924, Slice technique 1929, ATP 1930, Deoxyribose 1933, Glycolytic scheme
1933-43	Warburg theory	1934-35, TPN, DPN (NADP, NAD) 1936, Homogenate technique 1937, Citric cycle 1939, Oxidative phosphorylation
1943-53	Convergence theory (Greenstein) Protein deletion theory (Miller and Miller)	1950, Alternative metabolic pathways 1951, 5' RN-tides from RNA 1952, Pentose cycle 1952, Active transport across membranes
1953-63	Catabolic deletion theory (Potter) Morris hepatoma lines (Morris) Minimal deviation concept (Potter)	1953, DNA structure 1954, 5'-Ribonucleotides in acid-soluble fraction 1956, Feedback 1957, Repression 1958, Cyclic AMP 1960, Cell hybridization 1961, Genetic code
1963-68	Altered feedback theory (does not imply presence or absence of somatic mutation) (Monod and Jacob) (Pitot and Heidelberger) Molecular correlation concept (Weber) Altered mRNA template stability (Pitot) Metabolic activation of chemical carcinogens (Miller and Miller) Tumor promoters as reversible gene derepressors (Boutwell)	1964, Selection of cell hybrids 1964, Hormone modulation of enzyme activity and synthesis in cell cultures 1967, Cell-free mRNA- directed enzyme synthesis 1967, Hormonal modulation of developmental enzyme formation

Table 11. (continued)

Period	Cancer Biochemistry	General Biochemistry
1968- present	Reconciling hypothesis Provirus as gene (Temin) Unbalanced retrodifferentiation (Uriel) Dysdifferentiation (Sugimura) Unbalanced blocked ontogeny (Potter) Altered gene expression (Weinhouse) Pleiotypic response (Tomkins) Pleiotropic controls (Weber)	1969, Regulated termination of gene transcription 1970, Reverse transcriptase 1971, Restriction endo- nucleases for specific sequences in DNA 1972, Complementary DNA using reverse transcriptase with purified globin mRNA

[a]After Potter, 1977.

The Enzymology of Cancer

Glycolysis of Cancer Cells: The Warburg Theory

During the 1920s, the predominant investigations of the biochemistry of cancer centered around the monumental studies of Otto Warburg. In 1930,
Warburg published his book on the metabolism of tumors, in which he demonstrated that, in a wide variety of benign and malignant neoplasms investigated, tumors of both humans and lower animals exhibited a significant if
not very high rate of glycolysis. Warburg's hypothesis, which was reiterated
in 1956, states that cancer cells originate from normal cells as a result of an
irreversible injury to their respiration, this injury to the normal cell being
compensated for in the cancer cell by increased fermentation (glycolysis).
Until 15 years ago there were very few, if any, exceptions to this generalization, although many normal tissues exhibited equally high and in some instances even higher rates of glycolysis than the vast majority of tumors
studied; examples are embryonic tissue, the retina, and the renal papilla. In
view of these findings, two questions have arisen that have never been answered
satisfactorily by proponents of the Warburg hypothesis. The first is the association of glycolysis with growth rate. A number of studies have been carried
out in many laboratories that demonstrate a reasonable degree of correlation
of glycolytic rate with growth rate of tumors in many systems. We shall come

back to this point in more detail later, but it is clear that glycolysis may be a secondary event as a result of the loss of control of cellular replication in most neoplasms. The second unanswered question is the validity of many comparisons between neoplastic tissues and the cells from which they arose. This takes us back to our original definition of relative autonomy, which, as stated, was relative to the tissue from which the neoplasm arose. Unfortunately, Warburg and later Greenstein attempted to generalize their findings to include all neoplasms. Today it is clear that comparisons of normal liver with highly differentiated hepatocellular carcinomas reveal little, if any, differences in the glycolytic capacities of the two tissues, although, as these neoplasms continue to be transplanted, they tend to increase their glycolytic activity. Earlier investigations in the 1950s demonstrated the existence of primary hepatomas with little or no increased glycolytic rate as compared with liver. Malignant lymphoblasts glycolyze at essentially the same rate as their normal counterparts, and it is likely that malignant teratomas do not exhibit a degree of glycolysis in excess of that found in embryonic tissues. Thus, in support of Warburg's original hypothesis, most neoplasms do have relatively high rates of glycolysis, but, just as we saw normal karyotypes in early neoplasia, normal glycolytic rates do exist in many neoplasms. Increased glycolysis may, therefore, be a characteristic of tumor progression, similar to the occurrence of many karyotypic changes in neoplasms.

The Convergence Hypothesis of Greenstein

Approximately two decades ago, the late Jesse Greenstein, author of *The Biochemistry of Cancer,* the next major text after Warburg's work on the biochemical characterization of neoplasia, proposed that the biochemical constitution of tumors tended to converge to a relatively common enzymatic pattern. Several authors, including V. R. Potter of the McArdle Laboratory, pointed out that the Greenstein hypothesis had not challenged that of Warburg but actually extended it. Warburg's ideas of convergence were limited to the area of glycolysis and respiration, whereas those of Greenstein extended to a number of enzymatic functions in the cell. Greenstein understood and realized the importance of using valid tissue comparisons: he was among the first biochemists to realize the importance of comparing liver with hepatomas, since they are relatively homogeneous cellular populations. In stating the hypothesis of convergence, Greenstein recognized the existence of exceptions to his theory, although perhaps not their importance in an understanding of the cancer problem in general. As we shall see later, the exceptions to the Greenstein hypothesis have become more numerous, especially in early neoplasia. Like the Warburg hypothesis, the Greenstein idea of the convergence of neoplasms to a biochemically uniform cell type is untenable in the light of modern-day studies. A number of neoplasms may be maintained by multiple transplantations in vivo in a phenotypically highly differentiated state. This has been shown both with experimental hepatomas and mammary adenocarcinomas. Thus the differentiated characteristics of many neoplasms may be retained, and such cells do not converge to a universally uniform malignant phenotype. Yet despite the numerous exceptions to Greenstein's hypothesis, just as with the Warburg concept, Greenstein's experiments and his ideas have served to open new areas of fruitful investigation.

The Deletion Hypothesis

Unlike the two hypotheses mentioned above, the deletion hypothesis, first advanced by the Millers more than 25 years ago, was not based on studies with many different neoplasms, but rather evolved from investigations on the production of hepatic cancer by the feeding of aminoazo dyes. The basic experimental observation was that the dye became bound in a covalent fashion to proteins of the liver of the dye-fed animal, whereas little or no dye binding occurred in the protein of the tumors ultimately produced. The Millers thus postulated that carcinogenesis resulted from "a permanent alteration or loss of protein essential for the control of growth . . . ." Later studies by Sorof and others indicated that the proteins to which the dyes were bound in greatest amounts comprised an electrophoretically slow-moving class termed the h_2 proteins. These proteins were found to be missing from the neoplasms that were produced by dye feeding. Investigations with highly differentiated neoplasms have now shown the presence of the h_2 protein(s), although still little or no dye binding occurred in this fraction. Furthermore, it is now clear that, for the covalent linkage between amine carcinogens and liver macromolecules to occur, aromatic amine carcinogens must be "activated" by N-hydroxylation and subsequent esterification as described earlier (Chapter 3). Thus the absence of the dye binding in the neoplasms may be the result of a difference in blood supply, an absence of N-hydroxylase, or both, or of some other unknown factor(s). Later studies by the Millers and Heidelberger showed that a completely analogous situation took place during skin carcinogenesis by hydrocarbons. A protein has been isolated from mouse skin that binds hydrocarbons in a direct relationship to their carcinogenic activity for the skin. Electrophoretically this protein has many of the characteristics of the h proteins of liver.

Although the exact structure of the protein-bound form of polycyclic hydrocarbons is unknown, the fact that many of the metabolites of the carcinogens are freed from proteins by treatment with Raney nickel indicates that they are bound to the protein through cysteine or homocysteine residues. On the other hand, the studies by Lin and the Millers have shown that the structure of the major polar dye adduct obtained from the livers of animals fed N-methyl-4-aminoazobenzene is identical with 3-(homocystein-S-yl)-N-methyl-4-aminoazobenzene. Despite our knowledge of the structure of the major polar dye adduct, the function of the protein(s) to which the dye is bound has not been totally elucidated. At least two reports have suggested that one major dye-binding protein is alcohol dehydrogenase. This has been contested by Sorof and his co-workers. Another protein proposed as one of the principal cytoplasmic liver proteins that bind azo dye carcinogens is ligandin, a protein capable of binding numerous compounds including heme, steroids, and bile acids as well as a variety of carcinogens. This protein also has enzymatic activity catalyzing the conjugation of glutathione with a wide range of electrophilic compounds.

About 10 years after the original proposal of the deletion hypothesis, Potter suggested that the proteins deleted during carcinogenesis may be those identical or associated with enzymes involved in catabolic reactions, a view compatible with the Greenstein hypothesis as well as with some of the biological aspects of neoplasia, such as rapid growth. Furthermore, several experimental hepatomas demonstrated a complete lack of many catabolic reactions characteristic of liver. However, not long after the initial proposal of the catabolic deletion hypothesis, a series of highly differentiated hepatocellular carcinomas were produced in the laboratory of Dr. Harold Morris, and their chemical characteristics were studied by numerous investigators. These studies demonstrated that these neoplasms exhibited virtually all of the normal hepatic enzymatic functions investigated, and in several instances lacked any abnormal glycolytic capacity. These neoplasms also showed an extreme divergence in their biochemical phenotype, so that it was apparent that no two of these highly differentiated neoplasms were phenotypically identical. In fact, extensions of these investigations to primary hepatomas, mammary carcinomas, and even preneoplastic lesions have confirmed the ubiquitousness of this phenotypic heterogeneity.

The Minimal Deviation Concept

As a result of investigations with the highly differentiated Morris hepatomas, Potter proposed the concept of the "minimal deviation" neoplasm at the opposite end of the spectrum from those neoplasms conforming to the original Greenstein convergence hypothesis. Potter's concept was that some neoplasms were probably very closely related to or virtually identical with the initiated cell. The phenotype of such tumors deviated only slightly from normal with respect to their growth characteristics and exhibited relatively few abnormalities except those necessary for the expression of neoplasia. As these cells progressed, their deviation from the cell(s) of origin increased in the moderately or maximally deviated neoplasm. Thus the term "minimal deviation hepatoma" appeared to apply to a number of the Morris transplantable neoplasms. Although there has been some discussion of this concept in the literature, its correlation with both morphology and karyotype appears to follow the distinction among the degrees of differentiation of various neoplasms.

The Molecular Correlation Concept

Shortly after the demonstration of the existence of the minimal deviation hepatomas, Weber and his associates embarked on an extensive biochemical analysis of the enzymatic patterns of these neoplasms. These workers attempted to assemble the data into a modification of the Greenstein hypothesis but in direct relation to cell replication and the growth rate of the neoplasm. Thus, by the molecular correlation concept, certain enzymatic abnormalities seen in a class of neoplasms as compared with their cells of origin may be closely correlated with the growth rate of the tumor. Other functions, usually those more closely associated with the degree of differentiation of the organ, show little or no relation to the growth rate of the neoplasm. Weber's investigations have now been extended to include several different types of experimental neoplasms, numerous enzymatic functions, and specific metabolic pathways. A compilation of much of this data may be seen in Table 12.

However, the relation of these data to the process of initiation or to the initial transformation of the neoplastic cell is not clear. Just as in the case of the Warburg concept and that of convergence, it is more likely that the molecular correlation concept is a function of the progression of the neoplasm and that the metabolic changes seen may be related to this process, to the karyotypic abnormalities that occur, and to other changes secondary to the initial neoplastic transformation. Nevertheless, these data are quite useful for our understanding of the overall metabolism of the behavioristically malignant neoplasm and, as Weber has pointed out, for the potential that such data offer to the therapy of cancer directed at the metabolic changes seen in the metabolism of the fully developed malignant tumor. Therefore one may conclude that at present there is no evidence for a specific set of metabolic characteristics of the neoplastic state, but there is evidence that in the natural history of neoplasia there is progression of the neoplastic cell to a relatively uniform metabolism.

The Cybernetics of Cancer

With the advances in recent years in our knowledge of normal cells, it has been possible to study the biological characteristics of the relative autonomy of tumors from a chemical viewpoint. The hormonal control of enzyme activity and enzyme synthesis has now been well studied in many laboratories and is quite applicable to our understanding of the biochemistry of the neoplastic cell. A significant number of studies on the regulation of enzyme levels during hepatocarcinogenesis have been published, although no generalization can be made. With some carcinogens, the induction of certain hepatic enzymes by hormones is deleted or modified, whereas the feeding of other hepatocarcinogens has no effect on the same system. Clearly, the acute administration of a number of hepatocarcinogens markedly inhibits most hormonal effects on enzyme synthesis, but the relationship of these phenomena to the neoplastic transformation is as yet unclear.

Within the fully developed neoplastic cell, the feedback regulation of enzyme activity by metabolic effectors has in general displayed no dissimilarities between normal and neoplastic tissues. On the other hand, the environmental control of enzyme synthesis and degradation is clearly different when normal and neoplastic cells are compared in appropriate systems. Many of these examples have been demonstrated with the highly differentiated minimal deviation hepatomas and include deletion or modification of the regulation of the synthesis of a number of gluconeogenic enzymes as well as the dietary regulation of fatty acid synthesis and carbohydrate degradation. The one abnormality in control mechanisms that appears to be a characteristic of all hepatomas and is possibly applicable to other types of neoplasms is the loss of repressive control of cholesterol synthesis. This effect, which centers around the regulation of the synthesis of the key enzyme, hydroxymethylglutaryl-CoA reductase, a microsomal enzyme, has been described in both experimental and human neoplasms of the liver as well as in leukemic cells. Recent investigations, however, have questioned the significance of this generalization on the basis of the inability of neoplastic cells to accumulate and metabolize cholesterol itself and the fact that hepatoma cells growing in vitro do exhibit cholesterol repression of hydroxymethylglutaryl-CoA reductase. The regulation of drug-metabolizing

Table 12. Biochemical Functions Correlated with Growth Rate in Hepatomas[a]

Carbohydrate metabolism	Nucleic acid metabolism	Protein and amino acid metabolism	Other metabolic areas
Glucose synthesis: decreased	DNA synthesis: increased	Protein synthesis: increased	Polyamine synthesis: increased
Glucose-6-phosphatase	Thymidine incorporation into DNA	Amino acid incorporation into protein (alanine, aspartate, glycine, serine, isoleucine, valine)	Ornithine decarboxylase
Fructose-1,6-diphosphatase	Thymidine kinase		
Phosphoenolpyruvate carboxykinase	DNA polymerase		Urea cycle: decreased
Pyruvate carboxylase	Thymidylate synthetase	Decrease: S-adenosylmethionine synthetase	Ornithine carbamyltransferase
Glucose catabolism: increased	Deoxycytidylate deaminase	Enzymes catabolizing amino acids: Decreased	Lipid metabolism: decreased
Glycolysis	DNA nucleotidyltransferases	Tryptophan pyrrolase	Lipid content
Hexokinase	Ribonucleotide reductase	Serotonin deaminase	α-Glycerophosphate dehydrogenase
Phophofructokinase		5-Hydroxytryptophan decarboxylase	Butyrate to acetoacetate
Pyruvate kinase	DNA catabolism: decreased	Glutamate dehydrogenase	Respiratory activity:
Pentose phosphate pathway: increased	Thymine degradation		
C-1/C-6 oxidation of glucose			

130

Specific phosphorylating enzymes: decreased
Fructokinase and glucokinase
Fructose metabolism: decreased
Thiokinase
Aldolase

to CO_2
RNA synthesis: increased
Dihydroorotase
Aspartate carbamyltransferase
tRNA methylase
RNA catabolism: decreased
Xanthine oxidase
Uricase

Glutamate-oxaloacetate transaminase

decreased
Oxygen consumption
Mitochondrial protein content
Respiratory ATP production

Responsiveness to glucocorticoid stimulation: decreased
Response of gluconeogenic enzymes
Isozyme shift
High K_m isozymes: decreased
Low K_m isozymes: increased

RNA metabolic response to glucocorticoid stimulation: decreased

[a]From Weber, 1974.

enzymes is also defective in hepatomas, although not universally. It is of interest that, in contrast to the abnormal or deleted mechanisms for the regulation of specific enzyme synthesis exhibited by neoplasms in vitro, the model for studies of the molecular biology of the regulation of enzyme synthesis in vitro has been an inducible enzyme, tyrosine aminotransferase, in a hepatoma cell line in culture.

Biochemical Theories of Cancer in Relation to Abnormal Control Mechanisms

With the advent of the minimal deviation hepatomas as exceptions to the Warburg, Greenstein and deletion hypotheses, theories concerned with abnormalities in cellular regulation or "relative autonomy" were advanced. Potter proposed the feedback deletion hypothesis, suggesting that "in the minimal deviation hepatomas there has been a break in feedback control of cell division." Clearly, other control mechanisms were abnormal in such neoplasms, but in order to define the neoplasm operationally, growth regulation became the most significant of these abnormalities. On the other hand, it is not unlikely that the abnormality of the environmental control of growth in the neoplastic cell is basically the same as the abnormalities evident in the regulation of enzymes not involved in growth.

Within the last 5 years, the abnormalities in enzyme regulation as well as in growth control have been compared to the biochemistry of late fetal and early neonatal tissues, especially in liver. Such a correlation has been related to the isozymic profile of a number of enzymes by Weinhouse, Weber, and their associates. Potter and others have emphasized the potential importance of the analogy between neoplastic and fetal tissue. Their contentions are enhanced by the demonstration in a wide variety of neoplasms of the appearance of fetal antigens, a clear demonstration of major abnormalities in the regulation of genetic expression in the neoplastic tissues. Furthermore, in all instances the fetal antigens appearing in the neoplastic cell are not directly related to cell replication.

Differentiation and Altered Template
Stability in Neoplasia

A number of investigators have now demonstrated that messenger RNA molecules are stabilized for extended periods of time in the cytoplasm of mammalian cells. Furthermore, such stabilization of messenger RNA templates is an integral part of the process of cellular differentiation occurring in the development of the fetus. More than a decade ago Pitot proposed that an alteration in template stability of neoplastic cells could be the basis of the initial transformation event in neoplasia resulting in a "molecular mask" in the form of the neoplastic phenotype imposed on a normal genotype.

The details of the concept of altered template stability have given rise to a hypothetical cytoplasmic structure termed the membron. According to this model, the stabilization of messenger RNA templates occurs within differentiated mammalian cells through an association of the messenger RNA molecule with intracellular membranes, especially those of the endoplasmic reticulum. Differences in the messenger RNA template lifetime for four different enzymes in liver and three transplantable hepatoma lines have been documented. Furthermore, the lifetime of the messenger RNAs for any one enzyme in each of the hepatomas appears to be distinct. Therefore, altered template stability may explain the extreme diversity and phenotypic heterogeneity that are so characteristic not only of hepatomas but also of many other types of neoplasms, including mammary adenocarcinomas, myelomas, and thyroid carcinomas.

On the basis of the concept of altered template stability, the neoplastic transformation may be equated with an abnormal differentiation, resulting in a new phenotype. In this instance, however, the differentiation occurs in adult somatic tissues and is the result of the reprogramming of the expression of genetic information as a consequence of the interaction of the biological, chemical, and/or physical environment with the genome itself. Furthermore, the concept argues that the neoplastic transformation need not be solely the direct result of changes in cellular gene populations and chromosomal structure but may result from heritable cytoplasmic changes comparable to the phenomenon of differentiation.

Resolution of the Somatic Mutation and
Altered Template Stability Hypotheses in
Light of the Natural History of Neoplasia

It is obvious to any investigator in the field of oncology that the evidence for a genetic basis for neoplastic transformation is almost overwhelming, although entirely indirect. The fact that chemical carcinogens are mutagenic or may be converted to mutagens is important but not direct evidence for the genetic origin of neoplasia. The only direct evidence that neoplasms are genetically abnormal is that most malignant neoplasms exhibit karyotypic abnormalities in their later stages of development. On the other hand, the evidence for an epigenetic basis of neoplasia comes principally from studies of nuclear transplantation and the recent investigations demonstrating that teratoma cells inoculated into blastulas may exhibit complete reversion to the normal phenotype on development of the organism to the adult (vide infra).

These two apparently discrepant concepts may be reconciled by relating them to the natural history of the development of neoplasms in vivo. This concept is seen in Figure 22. The process of initiation, originally proposed by Berenblum, Boutwell, and others, is seen here to be the result of an altered differentiation resulting in a transformed cell with a perfectly normal genome but a heritably altered phenotype. In most neoplasms, however, this neoplastic phenotype tends to render the genotype relatively unstable, in that the natural history and tendency of such well-differentiated neoplasms if allowed to continue their growth is to develop chromosomal abnormalities and thus truly genetic alterations as compared with their cell(s) of origin. The development of aneuploidy may then be related to a basic membrane change which can affect the nuclear membrane such that the association of chromosomes or chromosomal components with this structure leads to the chromosomal abnormalities seen in aneuploid neoplastic cells. Obviously cells may be transformed directly into the promoted or progressed state without ever passing through the initiated state.

While this thesis is clearly far from proven, the recent studies of Mintz, referred to earlier (Chapter 6), and those of Gardner and his associates bear on this thesis. These investigators demonstrated that teratoma cells placed in blastulas develop as normal cells. However, Gardner extended these studies and showed that while teratoma cells exhibiting normal karyotypes developed in this manner, some aneuploid teratoma cells inoculated into blastulas developed into normal-appearing mice at birth, but these animals developed numerous teratomas and died shortly after birth. These studies indicate that neoplastic cells with normal genomes may, under suitable circumstances, lose their neoplastic phenotype and exhibit normal development, whereas some teratoma cells exhibiting obvious genomic abnormalities appear to have irreversibly fixed the neoplastic state. If these experimental results can be shown to have more general application in oncology, then Berenblum's original concept, which argued that the phenomenon of tumor initiation was irreversible although tumor promotion might be reversible, must be revised in that the opposite may be true in certain circumstances.

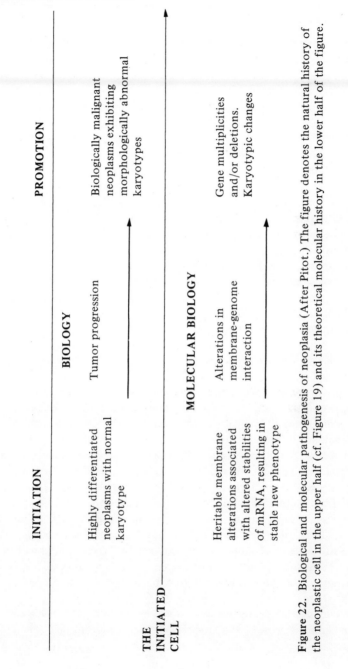

Figure 22. Biological and molecular pathogenesis of neoplasia (After Pitot.) The figure denotes the natural history of the neoplastic cell in the upper half (cf. Figure 19) and its theoretical molecular history in the lower half of the figure.

The Biochemistry of Transformed Cells In Vitro

Perhaps the best model in which to study the biochemistry of neoplastic cells in comparison with their normal counterparts may be found in systems of normal and transformed cells in vitro, when both are derived from the same tissue or cellular source. The first of such systems to be described, and still one of the best examples, was that of normal embryonic chick fibroblasts compared with these cells transformed by Rous sarcoma virus in vitro.

This system, as well as a number of other in vitro systems in which normal and transformed cells can be readily compared, has exhibited a number of interesting and relatively uniform biochemical characteristics. However, as with our earlier discussion, virtually all of the systems studied have been mesenchymal in origin. Thus any generalizations that have been proposed would be restricted to mesenchymal neoplasms, although, as we will see, certain conclusions reached with sarcoma virus and chemically transformed fibroblasts are applicable to some epithelial cultures.

Membrane Transport in Normal and Transformed Cells In Vitro

One of the earliest investigations of the biochemical changes accompanying transformation in vitro concerned various membrane functions. In particular, the transport of small molecules across the plasma membrane of transformed cultured cells was compared with this process in their cells of origin. In RNA virus-transformed cells there was an increase in the rate of glucose uptake concomitant with the first appearance of morphologic changes in the virus-infected cells. Furthermore, the available evidence indicates that this increase was dependent on the transformation process; e.g., hexokinase activity did not change at the time of transformation by the RNA oncogenic virus. The transformed morphology occurring in the cells after virus infection correlated with increased sugar transport, whereas the rate of sugar uptake in "revertant" cells was identical to that seen in the nontransformed cells. Perhaps the most conclusive evidence in support of this contention was carried out with temperature-sensitive mutants of Rous sarcoma virus. In these experiments, transformation of the cells occurred at $36°C$ but not at $41.5°C$. Similarly, the enhanced sugar transport was observed only at the permissive temperature ($36°C$); by shifting the temperature of the culture to $41.5°C$, one could decrease sugar transport to the level seen in the nontransformed cell. This change appears to be related to an increase in the V_{max} of the transport system and not to the affinity of the sugar for the transport system. More recent studies have indicated that the bound forms of hexokinase and of several other glycolytic and shunt enzymes increase significantly in Rous sarcoma virus-transformed cells. On the other hand, a recent study by Venuta and Rubin demonstrated that normal chick fibroblasts increased their rate of glucose transport up to 10-fold when the cells were starved with respect to glucose, although fast-growing normal cells doubled the rate of uptake of the sugar after starvation. Cells transformed with Rous sarcoma virus do not show any change in the rate of glucose uptake during starvation. Utilizing somewhat more sophisticated techniques, Bissell and her associates have demonstrated that the flow of glucose carbon into the intermediates of the tricarboxylic acid cycle and into amino acids in cultured chick embryo cells is unchanged after transformation by the Rous sarcoma virus. Unlike transformation of cells with RNA oncogenic viruses, SV40 virus transformation of mouse cells does not specifically enhance sugar transport. Transport mechanisms following chemical carcinogenesis in vitro have not yet been studied in detail.

Characteristics of the Surface Membrane of Normal and Transformed Cells In Vitro

We have already discussed the phenomenon of contact inhibition and its relation to tumor invasion and possibly tumor metastases. Obviously this phenomenon, which was first described in cell culture, must involve some alteration in the surface of the neoplastic cell. Attempts to study such alterations were rather unsuccessful until the demonstration by Burger of the agglutination of virally transformed cells in vitro by agglutinins (proteins) of plant origin (see Rapin and Burger); the source of the agglutinin was wheat germ. In contrast, the parent cells from which the transformed cells were derived did not agglutinate when specific plant materials were added to the medium. The purified material was found to be a glycoprotein having a molecular weight of approximately 18,000. This material was found to react with a number of neoplastic cells obtained from tumors growing in vivo as well as cells transformed in culture by chemicals, X-ray, viruses, or "spontaneously." In many instances revertant cells in vitro lost their agglutinability.

Since these earlier experiments, several other plant agglutinins have been found to affect neoplastic cells in a similar manner. In addition, some nontransformed cells also exhibit agglutinability, thus making the original generalization invalid. Furthermore, Burger and others demonstrated that treatment of normal cells with trypsin for very short periods of time rendered them agglutinable. This last experiment indicated that normal cells contained receptor sites for the plant agglutinins but that these sites were normally protected or covered over by some peptide components of the surface membrane. Furthermore, it was shown by Sachs and his associates that some variants of polyoma-transformed cells showed varying degrees of agglutination by another plant material, concanavalin A. More recently, Sachs' laboratory has demonstrated that normal fibroblasts in mitosis are agglutinated by concanavalin A as well as by the wheat germ lectin, whereas transformed fibroblasts in mitosis are not agglutinated by these lectins. The mechanisms of the agglutination of cells by plant lectins was initially thought to be concerned with covered or "hidden" sites. However, more recent evidence has demonstrated that lectins in the polyvalent form are capable of inducing a redistribution of lectin binding sites on the plasma membrane of the cell which becomes agglutinated. This is shown diagrammatically in Figure 23. Furthermore, under some circumstances the clustering of such sites may extend to the formation of a large mass of the sites on one portion of the cell surface that has been termed a "cap." The capping of such sites induced by lectins such as concavalin A has been shown to occur with some normal lymphocytes but not with neoplastic lymphocytes. On the other hand, many neoplastic cells, including some of the lymphoid series, can be shown to have clusters of binding sites induced by their interaction with concanavalin A. Other studies have demonstrated that in many cells in which agglutination is induced by these lectins, the microviscosity of the cellular membrane is increased in the neoplastic state. In the case of a lymphoid leukemia, Inbar and his associates have suggested that the loss in microviscosity is related to the cholesterol content of the membrane. By artificially increasing the viscosity of the plasma membrane of neoplastic lymphocytes, these cells appear to lose their neoplastic phenotype. Unfortunately, we are still not able to make the generalization that all neoplastic cells demonstrate an increased fluidity in their plasma membrane, nor is it possible to state the converse, i.e., that the plasma membranes of all normal cells have a greater intrinsic microviscosity than those of their neoplastic counterparts.

Becker has also demonstrated a differential lectin agglutination of fetal and malignant hepatocytes as compared with adult hepatocytes. The latter, even after treatment with protease, were not agglutinated by concanavalin A, whereas fetal liver cells and hepatoma cells were agglutinated by this lectin. Thus these epithelial cells appear to have different numbers of concanavalin A binding sites; this is not the case with the mesenchymal cells studied thus far.

In accord with the changes in lectin binding sites described above, biochemical studies of the surface membranes of normal and transformed cells

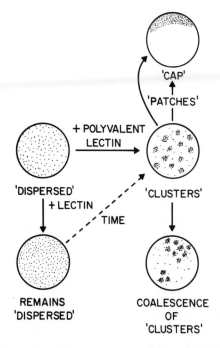

Figure 23. Pathways of ligand (concanavalin A)-induced receptor redistribution on cells. After ligand binding, initially dispersed receptors may remain dispersed or undergo clustering. The clustered receptor-ligand complexes may coalesce or form patches and eventually caps. (After Nicolson and Poste.)

in vitro have shown interesting differences. Surface glycoproteins and ganglio-sides of cells transformed by viruses, chemicals, and X-rays in vitro show significant but not necessarily common differences when compared with non-transformed cells cultured in vitro. In concert with these findings is the demonstration by several investigators of lowered levels in transformed cells of a glycosyl transferase involved in the synthesis of glycoproteins and gang-liosides on the surface membrane. A frequent finding in transformed cells in culture has been the absence or marked decrease of a cell-surface glycoprotein of molecular weight of about 250,000. This protein has been designated as LETS (large external protein that is transformation-sensitive). These findings, coupled with the suggestion that surface galactosyltransferase activity may be related to the process of cell-to-cell interaction, offer the possibility that in the near future we may be able to understand the mechanisms of contact inhibition, cell adhesiveness, and lectin effects on cells in relation to plasma membrane structure and enzymology.

Cyclic Nucleotides and Transformation In Vitro

Although it is more than 20 years since Sutherland and his associates discovered cyclic AMP, the possible role of this "second messenger" in the neoplastic transformation has been suggested only within the last decade. The studies by Pastan and his associates (see Johnson et al.), who demonstrated that the addition of cyclic AMP to transformed cell cultures resulted in an alteration in their morphology to that of normal, contact-inhibited cells with a lower growth rate, represented the initial findings in this now very rapidly moving area. It appears that the concentration of cyclic AMP in cells transformed in vitro is generally about one-half the concentration seen in corresponding nontransformed cells. Furthermore, in Rous sarcoma virus-transformed chick embryo fibroblasts, plasma membrane adenylate cyclase activity is reduced, and the K_m for ATP is significantly lower in normal cells than in the transformed cells. Pastan has suggested that these changes may be mediated through some modification of the plasma membrane by the viral transformation.

More recently another cyclic nucleotide, cyclic GMP, has been shown by Goldberg and his associates (see Hadden et al.) to vary with cell replication in a manner opposite to that seen with cyclic AMP — that is, cyclic GMP levels increase when lymphocytes are stimulated to replicate, whereas the levels of this cyclic nucleotide are decreased in starved cells, in which cyclic AMP levels increase. These changes in cyclic nucleotides have even led to the initial utilization of cyclic AMP in attempts to treat neoplasms in vivo as well as regulating the replication of their cells in vitro.

Perhaps one of the more interesting aspects of the cyclic nucleotides and transformation in vitro is the recent demonstration of a correlation between cyclic nucleotide concentrations and their effects on changes seen in the surface membrane. Pastan and his associates have demonstrated that in at least one strain of cultured cells low levels of intracellular cyclic AMP may be correlated with increased agglutinability by concanavalin A, whereas high levels of the cyclic nucleotide are seen in those cells exhibiting decreased agglutinability. Cyclic AMP also appears to affect the glycopeptide composition of the surface membranes of cultured cells, and the morphologic changes seen in cultured neoplastic cells after the addition of cyclic nucleotides are also associated with a reappearance of contact inhibition of growth in these cells.

In somewhat more differentiated cells, such as those of the neuroblastoma in culture, cyclic AMP addition to the culture actually regulates the morphologic differentiation of these cells in culture in that the addition of the cyclic nucleotide enhances differentiation of the neuroblastoma cells to differentiated neurons; this is accompanied by a decrease in cellular proliferation. In opposition to the effects of cyclic AMP, the addition of a nucleic acid base analog, 5-bromodeoxyuridine, to cultures of differentiating tissues (whether normal or transformed) inhibited morphologic differentiation of these cells. In certain neoplastic cells, especially melanomas, differentiated characteristics are lost when these cells are cultured in the presence of this analog. Furthermore, the tumorigenicity of mouse melanoma cells treated with the analog is markedly inhibited. However, after return of the cultured cells to media which do not contain the analog, normal differentiated characteristics and tumorigenicity reappear rather rapidly. One of the most interesting effects of this analog is its ability to "rescue" viruses from cells that are not producing the virus but that contain viral information within their genome. In this instance it would appear that the analog tends to enhance "differentiation" of the expression of the viral genome.

Plasminogen Activator(s) in Transformed Cells

Over three decades ago, tissue culturists were aware of the fact that certain neoplastic cells grown in vitro have the ability to lyse plasma clots rapidly. This observation has recently been re-evaluated, and Reich and his associates (see Unkeless et al.) have demonstrated that many cells transformed in vitro release a proteolytic factor into the culture medium that has the ability to activate plasminogen, an inactive precursor of the proteolytic enzyme, plasmin. The plasminogen activator of SV40-transformed hamster cells growing in vitro has been characterized as a protein of molecular weight 50,000. The production of this activator can be correlated in many transformed cells with the other characteristics that we have described above, growth in soft agar, agglutinability, and the suppression of tumorigenicity by 5-bromodeoxyuridine. Again, however, we are faced with the fact that the plasminogen activator is not produced by all cells transformed in vitro or in vivo. Thus, although activator production may be an important characteristic of specific transformants, it does not appear to be a ubiquitous characteristic of the neoplastic transformation. Unfortunately, at our present state of knowledge it is impossible to define the malignant transformation biochemically either in vivo or in vitro. Clearly, the phenotypic heterogeneity characteristic of highly differentiated neoplasms in vivo is a factor that was predicted by the morphologic variation described by pathologists during the past century. Although cultured cells offer the best possible systems for the delineation of critical differences between normal and neoplastic cells, as yet no generalizations applicable to all neoplasms have come from these studies.

References

F. F. Becker. Differential lectin agglutination of fetal, dividing-postnatal, and malignant hepatocytes. *Proc. Natl. Acad. Sci. USA 71* (1974): 4307.

M. J. Bissell, R. C. White, C. Hatie, and J. A. Bassham. Dynamics of metabolism of normal and virus-transformed chick cells in culture. *Proc. Natl. Acad. Sci. USA 70* (1973): 2951.

D. Burk, M. Woods, and J. Hunter. On the significance of glycolysis for cancer growth with special reference to Morris rat hepatomas. *J. Natl. Cancer Inst. 38* (1967): 839.

L. B. Chen, P. H. Gallimore, and J. K. McDougall. Correlation between tumor induction and the large external transformation sensitive protein on the cell surface. *Proc. Natl. Acad. Sci. USA 73* (1976): 3570.

J. K. Christman and G. Acs. Purification and characterization of a cellular fibrinolytic factor associated with oncogenic transformation: The plasminogen activator from SV40-transformed hamster cells. *Biochim. Biophys. Acta 340* (1974): 339.

J. K. Christman, S. Silagi, E. W. Newcomb, S. C. Silverstein, and G. Acs. Correlation suppression by 5-bromodeoxyuridine of tumorigenicity and plasminogen activator in mouse melanoma cells. *Proc. Natl. Acad. Sci. USA 72* (1975): 47.

P. L. Coleman, P. H. Fishman, R. O. Brady, and G. J. Todaro. Altered ganglioside biosynthesis in mouse cell cultures following transformation with chemical carcinogens and X-irradiation. *J. Biol. Chem. 250* (1975): 55.

T. H. Corbett and P. Nettesheim. Separation of multiple forms of protein-bound metabolites of the carcinogenic hydrocarbons 3-methylcholanthrene and 7,12-dimethylbenz(a)anthracene from several rodent species. *Chem.-Biol. Interact. 8* (1974): 285.

J. P. Greenstein. *Biochemistry of Cancer* (2nd ed.). Academic, New York, 1954.

J. P. Greenstein. Some biochemical characteristics of morphologically separable cancers. *Cancer Res. 16* (1956): 641.

J. W. Hadden, E. M. Hadden, M. K. Haddox, and N. D. Goldberg. Guanosine 3':5'-cyclic monophosphate: A possible intracellular mediator of mitogenic influences in lymphocytes. *Proc. Natl. Acad. Sci. USA 69:* (1972): 3024.

M. Hatanaka. Transport of sugars in tumor cell membrane. *Biochim. Biophys. Acta 355* (1974): 77.

C. Heidelberger. Chemical carcinogenesis, chemotherapy: Cancer's continuing core challenges. *Cancer Res. 30* (1970): 1549.

M. Inbar and M. Schinitzky. Increase of cholesterol level in the surface membrane of lymphoma cells and its inhibitory effect on ascites tumor development. *Proc. Natl. Acad. Sci. USA 71* (1974): 2128.

M. Inbar, Z. Rabinowitz, and L. Sachs. The formation of variants with a reversion of properties of transformed cells. III. Reversion of the structure of the cell surface membrane. *Int. J. Cancer 4* (1969): 690.

G. S. Johnson, R. M. Friedman, and I. Pastan. Cyclic AMP-treated sarcoma cells acquire several morphological characteristics of normal fibroblasts. *Ann. N.Y. Acad. Sci. 185* (1971): 413.

W. Levin, A. W. Wood, H. Yagi, P. M. Dansette, D. M. Jerina, and A. H. Conney. Carcinogenicity of benzo(a)pyrene 4,5-, 7,8-, and 9,10-oxides on mouse skin. *Proc. Natl. Acad. Sci. USA 73* (1976): 243.

J.-K. Lin, J. A. Miller, and E. C. Miller. Studies on the structures of polar dyes derived from the liver proteins of rats fed N-methyl-4-aminoazobenzene. II. Identity of synthetic 3-(homocystein-S-yl)-N-methyl-4-aminoazobenzene with the major polar dye P2b. *Biochemistry 7* (1968): 1889.

E. C. Miller and J. A. Miller. The presence and significance of bound aminoazo dyes in the livers of rats fed *p*-dimethylaminoazobenzene. *Cancer Res. 7* (1947): 468.

B. Mintz and K. Illmensee. Normal genetically mosaic mice produced from malignant teratoma cells. *Proc. Natl. Acad. Sci. USA 72* (1975): 3585.

G. L. Nicolson. Trans-membrane control of the receptors in normal and tumor cells. II. Surface changes associated with transformation and malignancy. *Biochim. Biophys. Acta 458* (1976): 1.

G. L. Nicolson and G. Poste. The cancer cell: Dynamic aspects and modifications in cell-surface organization. *New Eng. J. Med. 295* (1976): 197.

V. E. Papaioannou, M. W. McBurney, R. L. Gardner, and M. J. Evans. Fate of teratocarcinoma cells injected into early mouse embryos. *Nature 258* (1975): 70.

H. C. Pitot. Altered template stability: The molecular mask of malignancy. *Persp. Biol. Med. 8* (1964): 50.

H. C. Pitot. Neoplasia. A somatic mutation or a heritable change in cytoplasmic membranes? *J. Natl. Cancer Inst. 53* (1974): 905.

R. E. Pollack and P. V. C. Hough. The cell surface and malignant transformation. *Ann. Rev. Med. 25* (1975): 431.

V. R. Potter. Biochemical perspectives in cancer research. *Cancer Res. 24* (1964): 1085.

V. R. Potter. Biochemistry of cancer. In *Cancer Medicine* (J. F. Holland and E. Frei, eds.). Lea & Febiger, Philadelphia, 1973, p. 178.

A. M. C. Rapin and M. M. Burger. Tumor cell surfaces. General alterations detected by agglutinins. *Adv. Cancer Res. 20* (1974): 1.

J. Z. Rosenblith, T. E. Ukena, H. H. Yin, R. D. Berlin, and M. J. Karnovsky. A comparative evaluation of the distribution of concanavalin A-binding sites on the surface of normal, virally-transformed, and protease-treated fibroblasts. *Proc. Natl. Acad. Sci. USA 70* (1973): 1625.

S. Roth, A. Patterson, and D. White. Surface glycosyltransferases on cultured mouse fibroblasts. *J. Supramol. Structure 2* (1974): 1.

W. P. Rowe, D. R. Lowy, N. Teich, and J. W. Hartley. Some implications of the activation of murine leukemia virus by halogenated pyrimidines. *Proc. Natl. Acad. Sci. USA 69* (1972): 1033.

W. Seifert and P. S. Rudland. Cyclic nucleotides and growth control in cultured mouse cells: Correlation of changes in intracellular $3':5'$ cGMP concentration with a specific phase of the cell cycle. *Proc. Natl. Acad. Sci. USA 71* (1974): 4920.

S. Silagi. Modification of malignancy of 5-bromodeoxyuridine. *In Vitro 7* (1971): 105.

A. Sivak and S. R. Wolman. Classification of cell types. Agglutination and chromosomal properties. *In Vitro 8* (1972): 1.

G. J. Smith, V. S. Ohi, and G. Litwack. Ligandin, the glutathione S-transferases, and chemically induced hepatocarcinogenesis. A review. *Cancer Res. 37* (1977): 8.

S. Sorof, B. P. Sani, V. M. Kish, and H. P. Meloche. Isolation and properties of the principal liver protein conjugate of a hepatic carcinogen. *Biochemistry 13* (1974): 2612.

Y. Tokuma and H. Terayama. Isolation of carcinogenic aminazo dye-binding protein and its identification as alcohol dehydrogenase. *Biochem. Biophys. Res. Commun. 54* (1973): 341.

J. C. Unkeless, A. Tobia, L. Ossowski, J. P. Quigley, D. D. Rifkin, and E. Reich. An enzymatic function associated with transformation of fibroblasts by oncogenic viruses. I. Chick embryo fibroblast cultures transformed by avian RNA tumor viruses. *J. Exp. Med. 137* (1973): 85.

S. Venuta and H. Rubin. Effects of glucose starvation on normal and Rous sarcoma virus-transformed chick cells. *J. Natl. Cancer Inst. 54* (1975): 395.

O. Warburg. On the origin of cancer cells. *Science 123* (1956): 309.

G. Weber. Molecular correlation concept. In *The Molecular Biology of Cancer* (H. Busch, ed.). Academic, New York, 1974, p. 487.

S. Weinhouse and T. Ono. *Isozymes and enzyme regulation in cancer.* Gann Monograph 13, University of Tokyo Press, Tokyo, 1972.

11

The Host-Tumor Relationship:
Nutritional and Hormonal Factors

One must always remember in considering neoplasia, defined as we have in these chapters, that one is dealing with two entities, the host and the tumor. Each is independent and yet in many ways dependent on the other. The neoplasm is dependent on the host for its blood supply and other supporting tissues, whereas the host is dependent on the viability and subject to the nutritional requirements of the tumor for maintenance of the internal milieu of the organism.

It is quite apparent in oncology that this relationship of host to tumor and vice versa is perhaps the major factor in the clinical symptomatology seen in patients with cancer. According to the late Jesse Greenstein, "the host-tumor relationship is the key to the cancer problem." With the rapid advances in our knowledge of mechanisms in pathobiology, the problem of the host-tumor relationship has been considerably de-emphasized. However, this problem is as significant today as it has ever been in the past.

Nutritional Aspects of
Host-Tumor Relationships

It is not unusual for humans and lower animals with advanced cancer to lose weight and become emaciated even to the point that the host appears to die of starvation rather than as a result of any specific effects of the neoplasm itself. After the neoplasm reaches a substantial size within the host, it continues to grow regardless of the nutritional and hormonal needs of the host organism. In some experimental animals, body growth ceases when the neoplasm becomes grossly demonstrable; thereafter total body weight remains essentially constant while the neoplasm continues to increase in size and cell number. Finally, a significant decrease in body weight occurs although the neoplastic cells continue to replicate. In animals this latter phase may be correlated with the involution of the thymus.

During the phase of host weight loss a syndrome occurs in humans and animals that has been termed cachexia. This phenomenon has been defined by Costa as "the sum of those effects produced by neoplasms in the host, which are not the immediate result of mechanical interferences with recognizable structures." In humans, cachexia is characterized by weakness, anorexia, depletion of host components such as lipid and protein, electrolyte and water abnormalities, and a progressive fading of vital functions. The exact mechanism of this phenomenon is not understood completely, but many aspects of it have been studied both experimentally and in the clinic to the extent that certain phases of tumor cachexia are now better understood. Specifically, cachectic animals retain water as well as sodium and nitrogen. In addition, in many rapidly growing neoplasms there is an excessive production of lactate, presumably because of the relatively high glycolytic rate of the neoplasm. The host utilizes this material through gluconeogenesis. Many of these characteristics can be explained on the basis of hyperadrenocorticism, with an excessive production of cortisone as well as deoxycorticosteroids. Whether cachexia is simply a part of the well-known "stress" response or something relatively unique in response to the parasitic growth and metabolism of tumors remains to be determined.

One of the components of cachexia that has been described in both animals and humans is the progressive decrease in carcass lipids, especially during the later states of cachexia. The exact reason for this loss of carcass lipid is not clear; however, it may be related to the greater caloric expenditure characteristically seen in tumor-bearing animals, especially during the period of weight loss and tumor growth. As might be expected, hyperlipemia (excess lipid in the blood) is quite characteristically seen in advanced cancer; but usually ketosis or ketonuria, i.e., acetone and related compounds in the blood and urine, does not accompany the hyperlipemia. As might be expected with the rapid utilization of fat, the liver, especially with the added burden of gluconeogenesis, may be unable to metabolize the incoming lipid, and thus a fatty liver develops. This latter phenomenon has been especially noted in carcinoma of the breast.

The presence of a neoplasm can seriously affect metabolism in the tissues of the host. In addition to the local effects the malignant tumors have as a result of invasion, they also have general effects on the organism, the extent varying widely with the particular type of neoplasm involved. It appears that a neoplasm both concentrates metabolites to the detriment of the host and releases substances into the circulation that produce structural and functional changes in the tissues of the host. The tumor acts on the tissues of the host in two ways: first, by drawing on nutrients in competition with the host, and second, by depressing certain functions in the host tissues. Figure 24 shows some of the more frequently encountered effects of tumors on the protein metabolism of the host.

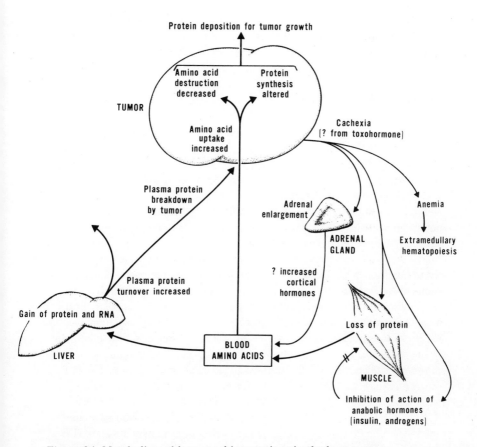

Figure 24. Metabolic and hormonal interactions in the host-tumor relationship.

Protein Metabolism and Tumor Growth

As might be expected of a rapidly growing tissue, tumor cells under both in vitro and in vivo conditions have been shown to have a high capacity for concentrating amino acids. Furthermore, tumor-bearing animals fed a protein-containing diet were actually observed to excrete less nitrogen and consequently appeared to be in a more positive nitrogen balance than controls without neoplasms. This is also true of human patients with advanced cancer. In animal experiments, analysis of the tumors showed them to contain more nitrogen than was retained during the experimental period. Thus, part of the tumor protein must have been obtained at the expense of the tissues of the host. This ability of the tumor to draw directly on its host tissue proteins is also illustrated by the observation that tumor growth in animals maintained on a protein-free diet was still about three-quarters of the rate observed in protein-fed animals. Observations such as these in both humans and animals have led investigators, especially Mider, to describe the growing tumor as a *nitrogen trap.*

Although the original studies leading to the concept of the nitrogen trap were carried out with only a few neoplasms, there is substantial reason to believe that the concept is applicable to many forms of cancer. Some neoplasms appear to have special types of nitrogen traps in the form of enzymatic capacities for the selective degradation of essential amino acids. When such a circumstance is present, the host becomes deficient in an essential amino acid, while the neoplasm still retains its ability to synthesize protein and to grow. This latter capacity undoubtedly is associated with the relative autonomy characteristic of all neoplasms, but other factors appear to play a role as well. Specifically, many neoplasms, especially those exhibiting relatively rapid growth, as would occur during the process of cachexia, have a decidedly greater ability to concentrate many, if not most, amino acids within their cells. However, other workers have demonstrated that shortly after the administration of a labeled amino acid, the "pools" of amino acids within various normal tissues are labeled to a much greater extent than those in the neoplastic tissue. Recently the interpretation of these data has become rather difficult in view of the studies by Khairallah and his associates, demonstrating that the amino acid pool utilized for protein synthesis is different from that of the pools of amino acids measured by standard techniques. Some years ago Busch and his associates showed that when labeled amino acids were administered to animals in the form of proteins such as albumin, tumor proteins were found to have a much greater specific activity than any in non-neoplastic tissue, suggesting that the amino acids in the form of proteins are better substrates for protein synthesis in neoplasms and that perhaps tumors have a selective advantage in extracting whole proteins from the bloodstream. Although this latter supposition has never been adequately studied, it is a well-known fact that patients and animals with large or rapidly growing neoplasms exhibit hypoalbuminemia.

The amino acid requirements of tumors do not appear to differ very significantly from those of normal tissues, other than nutritional requirements apparently associated with growth and possible specific abnormalities seen in certain neoplasms. A peculiarity of tumor nutrition has recently been exploited therapeutically by the use of the enzyme, *asparaginase,* to treat certain leukemias, wherein the tumor cells themselves require the amino acid asparagine for growth and survival. The use of this enzyme to deplete the host of a specific amino acid that apparently does not significantly compromise normal tissue metabolism differs somewhat from previous studies, in which diets missing certain amino acids were fed in an attempt to determine the effect of nutritional deficiencies on tumor growth. In the case of the latter attempts, very little effect was noted unless the neoplasm was very small or extremely slow-growing. More recently, attempts have also been carried out with enzymes that selectively degrade other amino acids, such as phenylalanine and methionine, in experimental systems. However, unlike the asparaginase system, the amino acids degraded by these enzymes are essential for normal cells in general, and, although inhibition of tumor growth was demonstrated, such preparations have not come into clinical use. Furthermore, comparable experiments have been attempted with amino acid-deficient or -limited diets, again with variable results. On the other hand, the use of vitamin-deficient diets has received some attention, especially since at least one vitamin analog, methotrexate (an analog of folic acid), is routinely used in clinical chemotherapy. In this instance it has been demonstrated that, in experimental animals, the drug is more effective when folic-acid deficient diets are fed. Patients receiving methotrexate must also be carefully monitored to ensure that the drug therapy, while combating neoplastic growth, does not produce a folic acid deficiency in the tumor-bearing host. Attempts have also been made to utilize various nutritional regimens to enhance therapeutic protocols, but it is clear that much work must be done yet in the study of the effects of host nutrition on the host-tumor relationship.

Humoral Factors and Serum Changes in Cancer

In addition to the peculiar metabolic effects of the tumor on the host, as evidenced by the need of the tumor for the uptake of amino acids as well as other metabolites, neoplasms also are capable of giving off various materials into the bloodstream that have effects on the host. One of the most widely studied of these is the so-called "toxohormone." It was noted some years ago that animals bearing neoplasms showed a markedly depressed level of the enzyme, catalase, in liver. Various purification techniques and studies demonstrated that certain low molecular weight protein-like compounds in the serum were apparently responsible for this lowering of catalase activity. Furthermore, these materials could be extracted from both animal and human tumors, and, in some instances, humans with far-advanced cancer showed low liver catalase. Normal tissues contained some, but very low, levels of this material. However, the entire issue of the significance of toxohormone in tumor-host relationships has recently been questioned by studies that indicate that only those tumors containing bacteria possess toxohormone-like substances. On the other hand, some relatively recent investigations by Japanese workers have demonstrated an inhibition of catalase by nucleotides, a fact that may throw a new light on an old question.

Another physiological finding associated with neoplastic diseases is that of anemia. A number of cases of anemia seen in cancer patients may be associated with peculiar immunologic effects. On the other hand, some anemias associated with cancer appear to be caused by the tumor's chemical interference with the erythropoietic process. One of the mechanisms for such a phenomenon is in all likelihood the nutritional demand by the tumor for key metabolites such as purines and folates. In addition, there is some evidence that neoplasms affect iron metabolism in the tumor-bearing host. Serum iron levels may be lower than normal in such organisms, and kinetic studies have shown that experimental neoplasms take up radioactive iron much more efficiently than do normal tissues, even liver.

While some studies have suggested that growth-promoting factors may be found in neoplastic tissue, it has also been demonstrated that during the latter phases of cachexia, liver regeneration is inhibited in the tumor-bearing host, possibly because of factors produced by the neoplasm.

In addition to hormonal factors produced by tumors, tumor growth appears to alter the enzyme and protein picture in blood proteins. Specifically, many neoplasms are accompanied by an increase in normal and/or the appearance of new serum globulins. These proteins are glycoproteins, a number of which appear to be in the slow-moving α_2-globulin electrophoretic class; these proteins appear in the plasma in response to wound repair as well as regeneration. The synthesis of these glycoproteins appears to be mediated by the adrenal cortex and thus is possibly related to the "stress" response or the mechanisms of cachexia. In addition, there is some suggestion that these glycoproteins may become associated with the surface of neoplastic cells, thereby affecting the antigenicity of the tumor cells as well as the entire immunologic response of the host to the neoplasm.

In addition to these findings, many neoplasms appear to "leak" enzymes into the serum. Acid phosphatase in the serum of patients with cancer of the prostate has been utilized in the diagnosis of this disease. Many neoplasms, especially one in rodents caused by a virus, may be accompanied by increased levels of serum lactate dehydrogenase. Many experimental hepatocellular carcinomas, while having lost the ability to secrete albumin into the serum, appear to have gained an ability to leak or secrete enzymes such as transaminases into the serum. Although changes resulting from the leakage of enzymes by tumors have found some use diagnostically, the mechanism is still unknown.

Hormonal Interactions in the Host-Tumor Relationship

The Effect of the Host on the Neoplasm

Partially by way of review and also as an introduction to the endocrine relationships in the interaction of the host and the tumor, we can consider the effect of the host environment on the growth of the neoplasm. Furth and many others have demonstrated experimentally that certain types of neoplasms will exist only in animals possessing very high levels of circulating hormones of the type to which the cell of origin of the neoplasm responds. Such examples in experimental oncology include thyroid neoplasms that exist only in animals possessing very high levels of thyrotropin as a result of direct administration of the hormones or of an endogenous source such as a thyrotropin-secreting neoplasm of the pituitary. Furth has defined a truly hormonally dependent tumor as "a normal tissue growing in an abnormal host." In addition, the normal feedback mechanism between the pituitary, hypothalamus, and receptor cell (in this case the thyroid) may be disrupted by removal of the receptor cell whose product normally represses production of the tropic hormone by the pituitary (Figure 9). Theoretically, a neoplasm of any of the receptor cells such as thyroid, testes, ovary, adrenal cortex, or mammary gland may produce a "dependent" neoplasm if the feedback effect is eliminated or if a source of excessive tropic hormone occurs in the cell's environment. In actual fact, in the human, it is doubtful whether such examples exist, although there are a few theoretical possibilities such as the "lateral aberrant thyroid" in patients who had been subjected to total thyroidectomy. On the other hand, the placenta may be considered a dependent tumor, being maintained only in the "abnormal" hormonal environment of the pregnant woman.

Continued proliferation of dependent or conditioned cells can lead to a gradual progression in proliferative vigor as a result either of environment (host)- induced modification of cells or of a natural selection of a more aggressive cell type. Such neoplasms can now exist in the host even in the absence of the tropic hormone or environmental stimulus, albeit at relatively low growth rates in many instances. Such neoplasms are termed "hormonally responsive" tumors and are exemplified by such neoplasms as carcinoma of the prostate or of the breast, since castration or treatment with hormones affects the growth rate of many of these neoplasms quite substantially. Less often, hormone-responsive tumors give rise to nonresponsive or "reversely responsive" variants, the original inhibitor becoming a stimulant of the tumor cell in the latter case. Although the latter situation is rare, it may be brought about by therapy in man and has also been shown to develop in experimental situations. Finally, responsive tumors may progress to an "autonomous" neoplasm, in which hormones have little if any effect on its growth rate. The natural history in humans of endocrine neoplasms is a progression from the responsive to the autonomous stage.

Hormonal Effects of Neoplasms on the Host

General Effects Possible
with Most Neoplasms

In many terminal cancer patients there occurs an adrenocortical hyperplasia. It has been suggested that this response, which may be the result of chronic stress, leads to an increased elaboration of corticosteroids, which act to cause an increase in gluconeogenesis, especially in the liver, with a resultant nitrogen loss by normal tissues. In many terminal cancer patients, hypoglycemia occurs, possibly as a result of the marked utilization of glucose by the extensive mass of neoplastic tissues. Hypoglycemia due to increased elaboration of insulin or insulin-like substances is considered later.

In a number of experimental situations, neoplasms have been shown to produce materials that cause effects in other organs, such as decreased or increased enzyme activities, but the molecular structure or characteristics of such materials or mediators are largely unknown.

Functional Neoplasms
of Endocrine Tissue

Neoplastic classification	Hormone elaborated by tumor	Clinical findings
Interstitial cell tumor of testis	Androgens	Masculinization
Thecagranulosa cell tumor of ovary	Estrogens	Feminization
Acidophilic adenoma of pituitary	Somatotrophic hormone	Pituitary gigantism or acromegaly
Chromophobe adenoma of pituitary	Thyrotropin	Hyperthyroidism
Adrenocortical adenoma	Aldosterone	Conn's syndrome
Adrenocortical adenoma	Cortisone	Cushing's syndrome
Phaeochromocytoma	Adrenalin or noradrenalin	Paroxysmal hypertension
Medullary carcinoma of thyroid	Calcitonin, prostaglandins	Hypocalcemia, diarrhea
Thyroid adenoma	Thyroxine	Graves' disease
Parathyroid adenoma	Parathormone	Hyperparathyroidism
Islet cell adenoma	Insulin	Paroxysmal hypoglycemia
Islet cell adenoma	Gastrin	Zollinger-Ellison syndrome, peptic ulceration
Renal cell carcinoma	Erythropoietin	Polycythemia
Carcinoid	Serotonin	Carcinoid syndrome

The above list gives a number of neoplasms arising from endocrine tissues that produce the hormones normally elaborated by their cell or origin. In most instances the production of the hormone shows essentially no environmental regulation by the host. On the other hand, there are now specific instances where such regulation does still occur, such as in the production of calcitonin by medullary carcinoma of the thyroid. In this example, calcitonin secretion by the tumor can be regulated by the administration of calcium, glucagon, or hypocalcemic agents.

Somewhat like the pituitary, neoplasms of the islet cells of the pancreas demonstrate a spectrum of hormone production (Figure 25). The β cell classically produces insulin and presumably is the neoplastic element found in insulinomas. The δ or α-1 cell of the islet produces gastrin, and neoplasms derived from this cell are responsible for the peptic ulceration of the stomach and duodeum found in the Zollinger-Ellison syndrome. In addition, other cellular species of the islets have been found to be producers of amines and the hormone, secretin. Neoplasms of these cells also produce an excess of such materials. Rarely, neoplasms of the α cells may produce glucagon, giving rise to hyperglycemia. In addition, more complicated syndromes involving multiple neoplasms of endocrine tissues occur, but are fortunately relatively rare, at least by our present frame of reference.

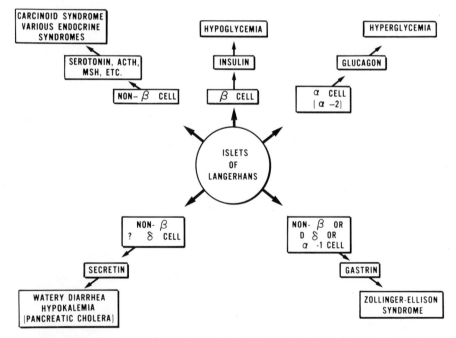

Figure 25. Spectrum of neoplasms derived from the islets of Langerhans of the pancreas. The hormones produced by each of the neoplasms is noted together with the syndromes resulting from excessive production of these hormones. (After Schein et al., with permission of the author.)

"Nonendocrine" Hormone-Producing
Neoplasms: The Paraneoplastic
Syndromes

In addition to the direct hormonal effects of neoplasms on the host as
seen in the case of functional neoplasms of endocrine tissue, within the past
15 years clinicians have come to recognize a number of specific syndromes
associated with neoplasms arising from nonendocrine tissues that are themselves capable of producing hormones or other factors that alter the normal
internal environment of the host. These syndromes or clinical pictures in patients having a neoplasm that elaborates some humoral factor that alters the
normal physiology of the host have been termed the *paraneoplastic syndromes*. While in some sense the effects of hormones produced by neoplasms
of endocrine tissue as noted above may be thought of as paraneoplastic, most
clinicians and investigators reserve this term for the specific syndromes associated with neoplasms of nonendocrine tissue that elaborate known and unknown factors producing definite pathophysiologic patterns in the host.
Some neoplasms produce protein or peptide components that have no hormonal action themselves but that compromise the overall function of the
host. Included in this class are lymphomas, myelomas, and thymomas that
produce γ globulin and related protein species with the attendant complications resulting from hyperproduction of such proteins. However, in these
instances, the paraneoplastic syndrome actually results from the production
of a protein normally elaborated by the cell of origin of the neoplasm.

In the case of neoplasms arising from nonendocrine tissues, a cell that
in its normal state produces no hormonal product may upon transformation
to the neoplastic state produce varying amounts of one or more, usually
polypeptide, hormones. Some examples of this phenomenon are considered
below.

The Ectopic ACTH Syndrome. This syndrome can no longer be considered a rarity, but is recognized with increasing frequency in many neoplasms
that arise in such diverse sites as lung, liver, kidney, parotid, and chromaffin
tissues. These neoplasms may produce a hormone that is biologically, physically, chemically, and immunologically indistinguishable from human pituitary adrenocorticotropic hormone (ACTH). Through its action on the adrenal
glands, this ectopically produced hormone can cause all of the symptomatology of Cushing's syndrome, a clinical picture of moon face, enlarged abdo-
men with linear streaking of the skin of the lower trunk, hypertension, and
salt retention. The production of this hormone is not suppressible by steroids, natural or synthetic. Occasionally it is associated with an increase in

melanocyte-stimulating hormone (MSH) or other polypeptide hormones apparently produced by the same neoplasm.

Other Examples of Nonendocrine Hormone-Producing Neoplasms. In addition to ACTH, carcinomas of the lung may also produce insulin, parathormone, thyrotropin, gastrin, MSH, and antidiuretic hormone. This is especially true in undifferentiated neoplasms of the lung, but it does demonstrate the extreme variability of expression for these polypeptide hormones that may be seen in a single biological class of neoplasms.

On the other hand, one may take a single hormone, such as insulin, and determine how many different types of neoplasms actually produce this polypeptide. In this case, production of the polypeptide or one having a similar action has been shown in neoplasms of the liver, cecum, exocrine pancreas, lung, and fibrosarcomas. Another example is parathormone, which has been found in association with neoplasms of the uterus, ovary, breast, kidney, and several sarcomas. In all instances, if the excessive production of the hormone can significantly alter the overall homeostasis of the organism, a clinical syndrome will be found in association with excessive hormone production or, as has been suspected in many cases, no specific syndrome will be noted but rather a number of symptoms that the clinician finds difficult to reconcile with other known clinical findings in the patient.

Other Effects of Neoplasms upon Body Systems. In addition to the known relationships among the effects of specific hormones producing the paraneoplastic syndromes, a number of effects related to neoplastic conditions have been seen in patients, but the exact mechanism is not clear. Some examples include acanthosis nigrans, a lesion of the skin that is usually symmetric, elevated, rough-surfaced, and hyperpigmented. Although there is some suggestion that this lesion is related to the production of MSH by neoplasms of the host, clinical experience has demonstrated that the majority of cases of acanthosis nigrans are found in association with carcinomas of the gastrointestinal tract. Arthralgia and hypertrophic pulmonary osteoarthropathy (forms of arthritis) have long been known to be associated with neoplasms affecting the lung and pleura. Many malignant neoplasms, especially carcinoma of the body and tail of the pancreas, have been associated with multiple venous thromboses (clots), and other neoplasms have been related to anemic conditions. A number of syndromes of muscle, nerve, and the neuromuscular junction in association with neoplasms have been described. Examples of myasthenia-like (weak muscles) syndromes have been reported in patients with various types of neoplasms other than thymomas. Polymyositis has been associated with neoplasms of the breast, cervix, gallbladder, lung, kidney, ovary, pancreas, as well as with leukemias and lymphomas.

Mechanisms of the Production of "Paraneoplastic Syndromes" by Neoplastic Cells. The student certainly must be aware that every cell within the mammalian body, with the exception of the egg and sperm, contains the same genetic information. Differentiation results from a selective suppression and expression of the genetic information available in the cell. There is significant evidence that neoplasia may, in fact, be a disease of differentiation, and the paraneoplastic syndromes can certainly be accounted for by such a theory. In essence, what may be occurring in neoplasms of nonendocrine tissues that produce hormones is the expression of genetic information normally suppressed in this specific cell type. This is borne out by the fact that the vast majority of nonendocrine neoplasms producing hormones elicit polypeptide hormones, and this requires the expression of specific components of the genome. Recently, however, some evidence has surfaced to indicate that small molecular weight hormones such as serotonin and prostaglandins may be produced by neoplasms such as the oat cell carcinoma of the lung and medullary carcinoma of the thyroid. Obviously the explanation for this is similar to that noted above but requires the expression of a larger component of the genome that is normally repressed in such cells. In addition, the production of hypothalamic releasing factors in several neoplasms has been demonstrated, with specific syndromes resulting from stimulation of the pituitary by the releasing factors produced by the tumor.

Undoubtedly these theories are by no means the whole story of the production of the paraneoplastic syndromes in humans. However, the clinical importance of such a phenomenon cannot be overemphasized in relation to the tumor-bearing patient. Rarely does the neoplasm itself by its growth and metastatic characteristics destroy the host. In almost all instances, death of the host is due to some, usually complex, host-tumor relationship that results in an irreversible imbalance of the internal environment.

Stromal Reaction of the Host to Neoplasms

In our discussion of benign neoplasms, it was demonstrated that the host may form a fibrous capsule around the neoplasm, apparently in an attempt to separate this growth from the remainder of the organism. The exact mechanism of stimulus of the production of this capsule is not clear. In some cases a portion of the capsule is probably also the result of collapse and degeneration of

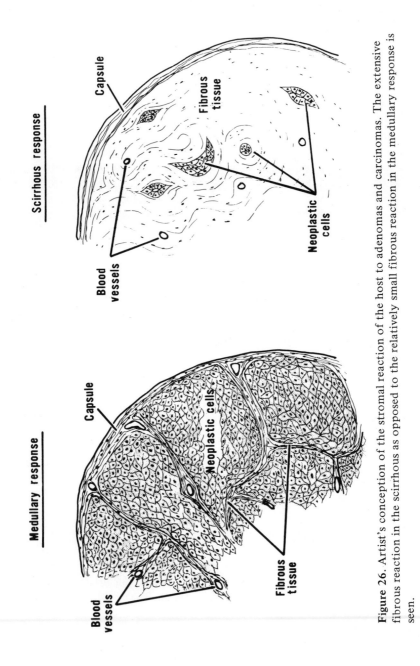

Figure 26. Artist's conception of the stromal reaction of the host to adenomas and carcinomas. The extensive fibrous reaction in the scirrhous as opposed to the relatively small fibrous reaction in the medullary response is seen.

neoplastic tissue. The host also supplies the blood vascular system for the nutrition of the neoplasm. The stimulus for this is not clear, but may be similar to the stimulation occurring during differentiation when the vascular supply to an organ is initiated. Recently a macromolecular complex has been purified from neoplasms that is capable of stimulating vascular proliferation in normal tissues. The blood vessels in a neoplasm are thus normal host tissue, not neoplastic. In a few rare instances the host stromal tissue, blood vessels, and supportive tissues may undergo a malignant transformation. The mechanism of this change is unknown at present. This may be seen rarely in certain neoplasms of the central nervous system as well as of the colon.

In certain neoplasms the host may react to the growth of the tumor in quite a peculiar manner. This is seen by the production of extensive amounts of fibrous tissue in response to tumor growth. Such a reaction has been termed a scirrhous reaction and the neoplasm, thus, a scirrhous tumor (Figure 26). This type of reaction may be seen in breast carcinomas and also in their metastases. Usually neoplasms inducing a scirrhous reaction in the host are limited to epithelial tumors that secrete glycoproteins and mucopolysaccharides. In carcinoma of the breast that metastasizes to the liver, the scirrhous reaction may be so severe as to compromise or even virtually destroy liver function. Tumors that possess very little scirrhous reaction have been termed medullary tumors when they are quite soft and composed almost entirely of the neoplastic tissue and its vascular supply (Figure 26). The terms medullary and scirrhous are quite commonly used with respect to cancer of the breast or other types of carcinomas.

References

J. Airhart, A. Vidrich, and E.A. Khairallah. Compartmentation of free amino acids for protein synthesis in rat liver. *Biochem. J. 140* (1974): 539.

C. A. Apffel and J. H. Peters. Tumors and serum glycoproteins. The "Symbodies." *Progr. Expl. Tumor Res. 12* (1969): 1.

S. B. Baylin. Ectopic production of hormones and other proteins by tumors. *Hosp. Pract.,* Oct. 1975, p. 117.

G. Costa. Cachexia, the metabolic component of neoplastic diseases. *Progr. Expl. Tumor Res. 3* (1963): 321.

E. D. Day. Vascular relationships of tumor and host. *Progr. Expl. Tumor Res. 4* (1964): 57.

L. J. Deftox, A. D. Goodman, K. Engleman, and J. T. Potts. Suppression and stimulation of calcitonin secretion in medullary thyroid carcinoma. *Metabolism 20* (1971): 428.

H. Ertl. A contribution to the clarification of the relation between tumor cachexia and thymus involution. *Oncology 26* (1972): 329.

J. Folkman. Tumor Angiogenesis. Therapeutic implications. *New Eng. J. Med. 285* (1971): 1182.

J. Furth. Hormones and Neoplasia. Thule International Symposia – Cancer and Aging. Nordiska Bokhandelns Forlag, Stockholm, 1968, p. 131.

J. Gold. Cancer cachexia and gluconeogenesis. *Ann. N. Y. Acad. Sci. 230* (1974): 103.

G. A. J. Goodlad. Protein metabolism and tumor growth. In *Mammalian Protein Metabolism*, Vol. 2 (H. N. Munro, ed.). Academic, New York, 1969, p. 415.

T. C. Hall. Oncocognitive autoimmunity and other paraneoplastic syndromes yet to be described. *Ann. N. Y. Acad. Sci. 230* (1974): 565.

C. R. Hamilton, L. C. Adams, and F. Maloof. Hyperthyroidism due to thryotropin-producing pituitary.chromophobe adenoma. *New Eng. J. Med. 283* (1970): 1077.

J. D. Hardy. On the cause of death in cancer. *Surg. Clin. N. A. 42* (1962): 305.

A. Herzfeld and O. Greengard. The dedifferentiated pattern of enzymes in livers of tumor-bearing rats. *Cancer Res. 32* (1972): 1826.

Y. Hokama and E. Yanagihara. The reversible inhibition of catalase activity by nucleotides and its possible relationship to mouse liver catalase depression induced by biological substances. *Cancer Res. 31* (1971): 2018.

T. Horai, H. Nishihara, R. Tateishi, M. Matsuda, and S. Hattori. Oat-cell carcinoma of the lung simultaneously producing ACTH and serotonin. *J. Clin. Endocrinol. Metab. 37* (1973): 212.

R. F. Kampschmidt. Mechanism of liver catalase depression in tumor-bearing animals. A review. *Cancer Res. 25* (1965): 34.

A. B. Lorincz, R. E. Juttner, and M. B. Brandt. Tumor response to phenylalanine-tyrosine-limited diets. *J. Am. Diet. Assoc. 54* (1969): 198.

K. E. W. Melvin, A. N. Tashjian, Jr., C. E. Cassidy, and J. R. Givens. Cushing's syndrome caused by ACTH- and calcitonin-secreting medullary carcinoma of the thyroid. *Metabolism 19* (1970): 831.

E. T. Peak, I. K. Mariz, and W. H. Daughaday. Radioimmuno assay of growth hormones in rats bearing somatotropin producing tumors. *Endocrinology 82* (1968): 714.

W. G. Satterlee, A. Serpick, and J. R. Bianchine. The carcinoid syndrome. Chronic treatment with p-chlorophenylalanine. *Ann. Int. Med. 72* (1970): 919.

P. S. Schein. Islet cell tumors: Current concepts and management. *Ann. Int. Med. 79* (1973): 239.

G. W. Sizemore, V. L. W. Go, E. L. Kaplan, L. J. Sanzenbacher, K. H. Holtermuller, and C. D. Arnaud. Relations of calcitonin and gastrin in the Zollinger-Ellison syndrome and medullary carcinoma of the thyroid. *New Eng. J. Med. 288* (1973): 641.

Symposium on hormone-related tumors. *Cancer Res. 25* (1965): 1053.

H. R. Tyler. Paraneoplastic syndromes of nerve, muscle, and neuromuscular junction. *Ann. N. Y. Acad. Sci. 230* (1974): 348.

G. V. Upton and T. T. Amatruda. Evidence for the presence of tumor peptides with corticotropin-releasing-factor-like activity in the ectopic ACTH syndrome. *New Eng. J. Med. 285* (1971): 419.

J. P. Whitecar, G. P. Bodey, J. E. Harris, and E. J. Freireich. L-Asparaginase. *New Eng. J. Med. 282* (1970): 732.

12

Immunobiology of the
Host-Tumor Relationship

For some years it has been evident that the various tissues of organisms are antigenically different. This is certainly obvious to the biochemist, since each tissue has a relatively unique enzymatic content and thus might be expected to be antigenically distinct. However, a number of investigators have extended these observations and demonstrated that each tissue has what are known as "tissue-specific antigens." The tissue-specific antigen is operationally defined as that antigen (protein or protein-complex) that is not absorbed by antibodies to extracts from all tissues other than the one under question. Tissue-specific antigens may be of the soluble variety, thereby evoking reactions of the humoral type characterized by circulating antibodies and produced by B-cell populations, notably the plasma cell. The various types of antibodies that are produced by B-cell populations are seen in Figure 27. The most common antibody is that termed IgG and may be involved in many humoral reactions to antigens of neoplastic cells. IgM is a polymer of this structure, while IgA is usually a dimer of the IgG structure that is secreted by glandular cells. During secretion by the gland cell, an additional protein component, termed the piece, is added by the secreting cell. Many neoplasms of plasma cells (myelomas) produce large amounts of a specific antibody or part of an antibody of one of the types seen in Figure 27. It is from those neoplasms that produce a single protein species that the structures of the immunoglobulins was first determined.

Antigens, especially highly complex antigens such as seen on the plasma membranes of whole cells, may also stimulate a cell-mediated immune reaction by thymus-derived T cells. The developmental relationships between T cells, thymus-derived, and B cells, "bursal-system"-derived, may be seen in Figure 28. The use of the term, bursa, is derived from the avian organ known

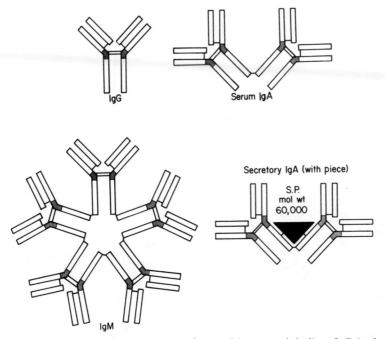

Figure 27. Comparative structures of several immunoglobulins. IgG is the more commonly found immunoglobulin, while IgM is the immunoglobulin characteristically formed as an immediate response to the administration of a new foreign antigen. IgA occurs in two forms, one in the serum and the other having acquired a small glycoprotein termed the piece after secretion from glandular tissues. The hinge region of the heavy chain (the longer bent structures in the figure) and the interchain disulfide bonds are also depicted. S.P. = secretory piece.

by this name which is the seat of production of all B cells in many avian species. In the mammal the exact counterpart to the bursa is not known, but it is believed to consist of many of the lymphoid structures of the gastrointestinal tract.

The relationships of T and B cells and their interaction with tumor antigens (AG) as well as macrophages may be seen in Figure 29. As shown in this figure, the tumor antigen may interact directly with any of three cell types involved: macrophages, T lymphocytes from the thymus, and B lymphocytes derived from the gut or bone marrow. With the possible exception of the macrophage, each of these cell types may be directly stimulated by antigen to produce either cells or products capable of reacting with the

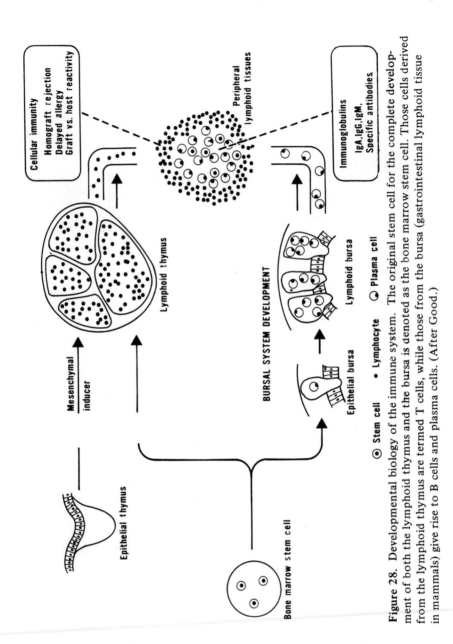

Figure 28. Developmental biology of the immune system. The original stem cell for the complete development of both the lymphoid thymus and the bursa is denoted as the bone marrow stem cell. Those cells derived from the lymphoid thymus are termed T cells, while those from the bursa (gastrointestinal lymphoid tissue in mammals) give rise to B cells and plasma cells. (After Good.)

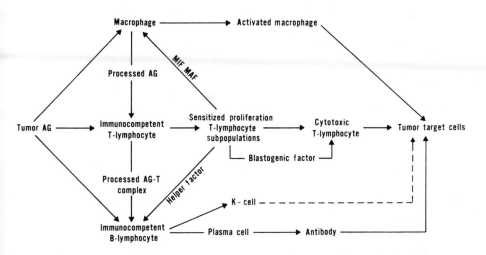

Figure 29. Pathways of cellular responses to a foreign or tumor antigen (AG). As seen from the diagram, macrophages as well as B and T lymphocytes are involved in the various processes. MIF, macrophage inhibitory factor; MAF, macrophage activating factor. (See text for further details.)

tumor antigen on the target neoplastic cell. However, a complex series of cellular interactions also exists, the major component of which is mediated by sensitized T lymphocytes and their subpopulations.

One of the major interactions that occurs is between T cells and macrophages, wherein the T cell immobilizes the macrophage in the presence of the antigen by releasing a soluble material, macrophage-inhibiting factor (MIF). The immobilized macrophage can then take up and process more antigen in the area, transferring this processed antigen to immunocompetent T cells, in turn creating still more sensitized T lymphocytes. These latter cells may also release a nonspecific macrophage-activating factor (MAF), which creates a cytotoxic population of macrophages that appears to distinguish malignant from normal cells, destroying only the former. Sensitized T lymphocytes may also release a helper factor that enables immunocompetent B cells to respond to antigens that they otherwise are unable to recognize. Macrophages may transport antigenic material that has already been processed by these cells. In turn, T lymphocytes can transport such processed antigens to immunocompetent B lymphocytes. These latter cells differentiate into plasma cells, which are the main producers of antibody molecules.

A population of cells, possibly variants of B cells and termed killer or K cells, is able to attack tumor target cells only after the neoplastic cells have been exposed to specific antibody. Proliferation and release of a blastogenic factor are not required for the development of individual cytotoxic T lymphocytes but are important steps in increasing the number of cells that can finally react with the tumor antigens. Some cells, not shown in the diagram, are formed from T lymphocytes and are responsible for "immunologic memory" and for an important set of feedback controls through which inhibitory subpopulations of these memory cells, termed suppressor cells, suppress the production of sensitized lymphocytes and antibody-forming cells.

Tumor Antigens

Just like normal tissues, neoplasms are antigenic. The critical question, however, is whether the antigenicity of neoplasms is different in any way from that of their cells of origin. Early investigations in this field with inbred mice and hydrocarbon-induced sarcomas showed that immunologic resistance of the host to the syngeneic neoplasm could be established, although no immunologic response could be obtained to spontaneously arising mammary carcinomas. As a result of these studies, Klein and his associates, utilizing whole animal experiments, were able to demonstrate that chemically induced and transplanted neoplasms evoke specific reactions of the cellularly mediated type (T cell) in recipient or host animals. The antigens evoking such reactions were termed tumor-specific transplantation antigens (TSTA). For demonstration of such antigens it was important to utilize neoplasms of recent origin, since serial passage through many generations caused neoplasms to undergo antigenic changes by mechanisms not totally understood but quite possibly related to the phenomenon of tumor progression with karyotypic alterations. The TSTA is a complex surface antigen, which is lost upon destruction of the surface membrane of the cell. Klein and his associates also made the interesting observation that TSTAs of chemically induced neoplasms were essentially unique to each neoplasm, while those of virally induced neoplasms were identical for each virus. Furthermore, it is clear that the TSTA of virus-induced cancers is quite distinct antigenically from the S and T antigens mentioned earlier in our discussion on viral oncology. Each tumor produced by radiation also appears to have its own unique tumor-specific transplantation antigen. Furthermore, the TSTAs of chemically or radiation-induced neoplasms were in no way related to the chemical or agent causing the tumor, since a single chemical could be shown to induce numerous primary neoplasms in one animal, each neoplasm having a different TSTA. The possible number of different tumor-specific transplantation antigens in chemically induced neoplasms is not certain, since no two neoplasms have ever been definitively found to possess the same TSTA when induced by chemicals or radiation.

Neoplasms arising spontaneously in animals fail to elicit a specific immunologic resistance in the transplantation tests in syngeneic animals. Occasionally a resistance reaction is found, but it is invariably weak, and some investigators argue that, because of this finding, spontaneous tumors do have TSTAs but that for practical purposes they are not sufficiently antigenic to stimulate specific immunologic resistance in the host.

Little is actually known about the chemical nature of tumor-specific transplantation antigens. However, they undoubtedly represent the cumulative antigenicity of a number of surface components of the cell, and this allows the host to recognize such a structure as foreign. In addition to the TSTA, some neoplasms have tumor-specific antigens (TSA) that are unique to the neoplasm itself. Thus melanomas have tumor-specific antigens that are unique to this neoplasm. These tumor-specific antigens evoke both humoral and cell-mediated responses within the organism. These antigens do not cross-react with antigens in other types of neoplasms or in normal tissues, with the exception of the cells from which melanomas arise, melanocytes. Similar tumor-specific antigens have been described for the neuroblastoma and for soft tissue sarcomas in the human. In both of these instances humoral as well as cell-mediated responses to these antigens occur in the host. One might also consider the T and S antigens induced by viral oncogens as tumor-specific antigens (see Chapter 4). As we shall see later, some of these antigens may play a role in the overall host resistance to the neoplasm.

In addition to tumor-specific transplantation antigens, a number of neoplasms contain antigens that are both different from and similar to their tissue of origin. An entire group of these antigens have now been classified as embryonic antigens, which are characteristic of the embryonic tissue of the adult organ from which the neoplasm arose. The best known example of this class is an embryonic antigen of the gastrointestinal tract, termed CEA; this has been found to occur in a large number of neoplasms of this organ or of related structures such as the pancreas, liver, and even lung. Recent studies have suggested that some of the viral antigens, such as the S antigen described earlier, may be related to embryonic antigens. In addition, as might be expected, some embryonic antigens also cross-react with antigens found in adult tissues.

Another fetal antigen, which has been described in the human and is now utilized for diagnostic and well as therapeutic purposes, is alpha-fetoprotein, an embryonic protein produced by hepatomas and several other types of neoplasms in the human, including those of the testes, pancreas, and gastrointestinal tract. In the case of both CEA and alpha-fetoprotein, the host produces circulating antibodies as its major response to these antigens in many but not all patients. Alpha-fetoprotein has also been demonstrated to occur in animals fed hepatocarcinogens prior to the demonstration or estab-lishment of hepatomas in the liver.

Immunosurveillance

Almost 20 years ago Thomas suggested that the host possesses a normal homeostatic cellular mechanism active in eliminating "nonself" antigenic components such as parasites, mutated cells, and neoplastic cells. This con-cept predicted that patients with immunodeficiency not only would be more susceptible to parasitic infections, but should be expected to be quite suscep-tible to the development of malignant disease. Later studies by Good and his associates demonstrated that this was so in that genetic defects of the im-mune system in patients usually rendered them highly prone to the develop-ment of neoplasms, although these neoplasms were almost always of cells from the immune system. Further substantiation of this concept came from the widespread therapeutic use of organ transplantation with associated chemical and radiologic immunosuppression in order to obtain reasonably functioning transplants in the face of the host immune defenses. As a result of a survey of such transplant patients, it has been shown that the incidence of cancer in such patients is approximately 25 times higher than in the nor-mal population. In one specific instance, that of reticulum cell sarcoma, the incidence of this neoplasm in patients who had been immunosuppressed for organ transplants is 300 times higher than in the normal population.

The recent discovery that a mutation in the so-called "nude" mouse results in virtually a complete absence of thymic development presents another system in which to study neoplastic growth in the absence of cell-mediated immunity. The cell-mediated response of such mutant animals is essentially nonexistent, yet the incidence of spontaneous carcinomas and neoplasms other than those of the immune system is actually no different from that of nonmutant controls and laboratory mice in general. On the other hand, if newborn nude mice are inoculated with polyoma virus, they develop on the average eight distinct neoplasms per animal, many more than a mouse with an intact immune system would develop under the same cir-cumstances. Therefore, the role of immunosurveillance in the host resistance to cancer, although undoubtedly important, is in all likelihood not the only factor in carcinogenesis; in many situations, such as with spontaneous neoplasms virtually lacking TSTAs, it may play only a minor role, if any.

Lymphomagenesis and the Graft vs. Host Reaction

As our knowledge of immunobiology has increased rapidly over the past several decades, a number of experimental systems that have potential direct application to specific disease conditions in the human have been developed. One such system has been the production of "runt" disease by inducing a graft vs. host reaction in rodents as well as in other species. The basis for such experiments was the demonstration that fetal and neonatal organisms did not develop an immune response to many foreign antigens with which the organism was challenged. Rather, the fetal and neonatal organism became tolerant to such antigenic species administered during these developmental stages, and thereafter repeated challenge with the same antigen invoked no immune response in the host.

The production of the graft vs. host reaction resulting in runt disease is outlined in Figure 30, wherein immunocompetent lymphoid and bone marrow tissue is removed from an adult animal that is genetically distinct from the recipient neonate. The cells from the adult survive within the neonatal animal because it does not produce a rejection reaction to the cells. However, the cells from the adult donor do react with the host tissues producing both humoral and cell-mediated responses. Such a reaction of the donor cells damages the host tissues eventually to the point of death. During this process the young animal does not grow — thus the term "runt" — and may also exhibit other changes of the skin, tails, ears, and internal organs. A similar condition may be produced in the adult by making the recipient tolerant to a small number of cells, insufficient to produce runt disease, and subsequently administering a large number of immunocompetent cells from the same donor to the original recipient when this tolerant animal has grown to adulthood. This experimental model is quite similar to many conditions found in the human under the general category of autoimmune diseases in which both humoral and cell-mediated immunity to the host's own tissues are produced by cellular populations within the host.

One of the most interesting phenomena from such investigations has been the description by Schwartz and the Gleichmanns of the development of malignant lymphomas in recipient mice undergoing a chronic graft vs. host

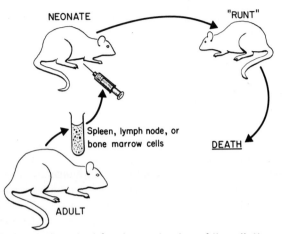

Figure 30. Classical method for the production of "runt" disease or a graft vs. host reaction. Immunocompetent cells from the spleen, lymph node, or bone marrow are removed from an adult animal and inoculated into a neonate. Since the neonate is immunologically deficient, it will not react to the donor cells, but the donor cells will react with the host tissues to produce a graft vs. host reaction and runt disease with ultimate death.

reaction. In this instance the reaction is produced by the injection of parental spleen cells into the neonatal offspring. The same sequence of events occurs as is seen in Figure 30, but the recipient now contains 50% of the genes of the donor. Thus the reaction is much milder, and most of the recipients survive and develop. However, later in life many of these animals develop lymphomas. These lymphomas may develop either from the original donor cells administered during the neonatal period or from the host cells. In theory one would expect that the marked stimulation of the donor cells might ultimately lead to their neoplastic transformation. However, it is known that lymphoid cells of the host proliferate quite extensively in the graft vs. host reaction, although the reason for this is not understood. It would appear that the lymphomas resulting from these graft vs. host reactions in genetically related animals are the result of chronic immunologic stimulation of lymphoid cells, although some evidence has indicated a role for oncogenic RNA viruses in lymphoma production.

In the human the association of autoimmune disease and lymphomas is now well recognized. Furthermore, certain types of lymphomas such as Hodgkin's disease may be related to immunodeficiencies in the host. The classification of lymphomas as to whether they are predominantly of B- or T-cell origin is now made possible by the immunologic distinction between these two classes of cells. It is of interest that the most common neoplasm developing during the graft vs. host reaction has been termed a reticulum cell sarcoma or "the Hodgkin's-like lesion of the mouse." Evidence to date indicates that such neoplasms are of B-cell origin.

Host Resistance to Neoplasia

In view of the fact that many neoplasms do exhibit antigens that the host recognizes as foreign, it should be theoretically possible to stimulate the host defenses to eliminate many neoplasms. In actual fact, however, this phenomenon does not occur. An interesting piece of evidence against the efficacy of minimal immunity toward early neoplasms is the so-called "sneaking through" phenomenon. This term was coined by Old, Boyse, and others to describe a situation in which medium-sized inocula of antigenic, chemically induced tumor cells were rejected in syngeneic recipients, while both large and very small inocula grew quite well. Although no definitive explanation for this phenomenon has been proposed, one suggestion is that a very few tumor cells fail to signal the immune response to their presence effectively. A delay in this signal may then allow the inoculated cells to establish themselves and to grow to a size too large for efficient destruction by the host immune system. "Sneaking through" can also be relevant to the two-stage phenomenon of carcinogenesis, whereby promotion facilitates the proliferation of the early neoplastic cells, although promoters do not appear to act by immunosuppression per se. However, the role of the "sneaking through" phenomenon is probably minor, if it occurs at all, in minimally immunogenic spontaneous neoplasms.

Blocking Factors

Since the early neoplasm does continue to grow and produce more antigenic material, it is important to consider mechanisms for the failure of the host to respond to this continued antigenic stimulus. An explanation has been proposed for at least several neoplasms, including the melanoma and neuroblastoma in the human. The Hellström's and their associates have demonstrated factors in the serum of patients with these neoplasms that are protein in nature and possibly contain antibody structures; these factors apparently prevent the action of sensitized T lymphocytes on the neoplastic cells. Such factors have been termed "blocking" factors and presumably are components that coat the surface of tumor cells and thus prevent the reaction of cellular immunity by sensitized T cells and killer cells. Although the molecular nature of such blocking factors is not understood at the present time, it is possible that they are actually antigen-antibody complexes associated with the surface of the tumor cell. In a significant number of neoplasms one can demonstrate the presence of large numbers of antigen-antibody complexes, which may actually affect the host in other ways, such as damaging the glomeruli of the kidney, where they are filtered out and inhibit the normal process of filtration by the kidney. Where there is extensive production of such complexes, they may actually deposit in perivascular areas and possibly contribute to the formation of a substance called "amyloid" with significant consequences to the health of the individual. A recent study has also demonstrated the presence of circulating fibrinogen degradation products in patients with advanced cancer. Some of these degradation products of normal blood clotting proteins have been shown to be immunosuppressive and thus may contribute to the relative immunologic paralysis of the advanced cancer patient.

An interesting immunologic response to oncogenic virus infections has been shown in the AKR mouse, which possesses an endogenous oncogenic RNA virus, the genes for which are present in all cellular genomes of the animal including the egg and sperm. As a result of the endogenous nature of the virus, for years investigators felt that the host was tolerant to the antigens of the virus. Recently Dixon and his associates have demonstrated that this is not true, but rather that the host produces antibodies to viral antigens. However, such humoral immunity is difficult to detect, since virtually all of the antibodies are probably associated with viral antigens. Therefore, the basis for persistent viral infection would be the result of a unique behavior of the endogenous virus itself in interacting with antibody to the virus produced by the host rather than of the immunologic hyporesponsiveness of the host.

Despite these difficulties, attempts have been made to treat human neoplasia by immunotherapy. In a theoretical vein, the most efficacious type of therapy would be to combine chemotherapy and immunotherapy, with the latter being effective against the cells remaining after massive drug therapy of neoplasms such as leukemia. The "sneaking through" phenomenon should not come into play in this situation, since the host's immune response to the neoplasm should be maximal. However, attempts to immunize with specific TSAs have met with virtually no success, and most clinical trials have been oriented toward a general and nonspecific stimulation of the immune response by the administration of BCG, a vaccine originally utilized against tuberculosis. This material, which consists of live attenuated tubercle bacilli, has been given subcutaneously or even directly into the neoplasm in an attempt to stimulate host responses to destroy the tumor. In certain experimental systems this has been quite efficacious in combination with other types of therapy and occasionally even alone. Unfortunately, in some experimental situations, neoplastic growth has been enhanced after the administration of BCG to the host. The mechanism of this enhancement is unknown at the present time but is undoubtedly complicated, possibly involving blocking factors and a partial immunologic paralysis of the host. In humans, BCG has been utilized in combination with chemotherapy in cases of acute leukemia, especially in children, and also with certain solid tumors, such as melanoma in the adult. However, it is clear that immunotherapy and the immunologic response of the host to neoplasms, as well as the chemistry of the antigens of cancer cells, are far from being understood at this time.

Infectious Complications of
Neoplastic Disease

One of the characteristics of advanced cancer, especially neoplasms of the immune system, is a decrease in the host resistance to various infectious agents. Specifically, this phenomenon appears to have three characteristics: (1) a decrease in mature granulocytes, seen in several lymphomas and leukemias, may result in impaired phagocytosis; (2) an impaired cell-mediated immune response, commonly seen in several lymphomas and leukemias, especially Hodgkin's disease; and (3) a decrease or alteration in circulating γ globulin of host origin, found in a number of lymphomas and leukemias, resulting in an increased susceptibility to bacterial infections. In addition to the natural loss of host immunity resulting from the host-tumor relationship, chemotherapy itself may result in a marked suppression of the host immune response, leading to a number of infectious complications.

Many of the infectious processes that occur in patients with advanced cancer or undergoing chemotherapy are the result of agents that normally do not cause disease in the host. Table 13 shows a list of those organisms that may cause severe infection in patients with neoplastic disease. The reader will note some familiar infectious agents such as salmonella (typhoid), tuberculosis, measles, and varicella (chicken pox). But most of the agents listed in the table are relatively rare causes of disease in the normal human. These latter organisms can usually attack only the individual whose immune defenses are compromised. This is especially true of fungi and cytomegalovirus, which appear to be ubiquitous in the human population but rarely cause disease in the immunocompetent host. Earlier we had seen that patients with

Table 13. Organisms Showing a Predilection for Causing Severe Infection in Patients with Neoplastic Disease

Bacterial	Fungal	Parasitic	Viral
Listeria monocytogenes Salmonella species *Nocardia asteroides* Mycobacterium tuberculosis Enteric bacteria	Canadian species *Cryptococcus neoformans* *Histoplasma capsulatum* Mucor species Aspergillus species *Coccidioides immitus* *Sporotrichum schenckii*	*Pneumocystis carinii* *Toxoplasma gondii*	Cytomegalovirus Varicella zoster virus Herpes simplex virus Vaccinia virus Measles virus

(After D. Armstrong et al., 1971.)

progressive multifocal leukoencephalopathy (PML) were found to have a papovavirus infection within the central nervous system. It is quite likely that the virus causes PML, but only in humans who exhibit significant immuno-suppression associated with lymphomas and other debilitating diseases. An interesting organism not listed in the table is *Clostridium septicum,* anaer-obic bacteria related to microorganisms causing gas gangrene. In some pa-tients receiving extensive therapy with resultant destruction of large masses of tumor, this organism has been found growing within the dead tissue of the neoplasm and has lead to complications in the therapy.

Thus the extensive growth of tumors, predominantly but not exclusively those of the immune system, results in significant loss of immune resistance by the host with the resultant danger of an "opportunistic" infection by a variety of agents. On the other hand, heroic measures of therapy by chemi-cals and radiation may also leave the host immunosuppressed and vulnerable to infection. In many instances it is this infectious sequel of cancer or its therapy that leads to the ultimate demise of the patient.

References

D. Armstrong, L. S. Young, R. D. Meyer, and A. H. Blevins. Infectious complications of neoplastic disease. *Med. Clin. N.A. 55* (1971): 729.

L. D. Berman. The SV 40 S Antigen: A carcinoembryonic-type antigen of the hamster? *Int. J. Cancer 10* (1972): 326.

P. J. Deckers, R. C. Davis, G. A. Parker, and J. A. Mannick. The effect of tumor size on concomitant tumor immunity. *Cancer Res. 33* (1973): 33.

S. O. Freedman. Carcinoembryonic antigen. Current clinical application. *Allergy Clin. Immunol. 50* (1972): 348.

G. Girmann, H. Pees, G. Schwarze, and P. G. Scheurlen. Immunosuppression by micromolecular fibrinogen degradation products in cancer. *Nature 259* (1976): 399.

E. Gleichmann, H. Gleichmann, and R. S. Schwartz. Immunologic induction of malignant lymphoma. Genetic factors in the graft-versus-host model. *J. Natl. Cancer Inst. 49* (1972): 793.

E. Gleichman, H. Gleichmann, and W. Wilke. Autoimmunization and lymphomagenesis in parent-F_1 combinations differing at the major histocompatibility complex: Model for spontaneous disease caused by altered self-antigens? *Transplant Rev. 31* (1976): 156.

R. A. Good. Disorders of the immune system. In *Immunobiology* (R. A. Good and D. W. Fisher., eds.). Sinauer Assoc., Inc., Stamford, 1971, pp. 3-17.

I. Hellström, G. A. Warner, K. E. Hellström, and H. O. Sjögren. Sequential studies on cell-mediated tumor immunity and blocking serum activity in ten patients with malignant melanoma. *Int. J. Cancer 11* (1973): 280.

G. Klein. Tumor immunology. *Transplant. Proc. 5* (1973): 31.

J.-P. Mach and G. Pusztaszeri. Carcinoembryonic antigen: Demonstration of the partial identity between CEA and a normal glycoprotein. *Immunochemistry 9* (1972): 1031.

C. F. McKhann and M. A. Yarlott. Tumor immunology. *Ca 25* (1975): 187.

L. J. Old, E. A. Boyse, D. A. Clarke, and E. A. Carswell. Antigenic properties of chemically induced tumors. *Ann. N. Y. Acad. Sci. 101* (1962): 80.

M. B. A. Oldstone, T. Aoki, and F. J. Dixon. The antibody response of mice to murine leukemia virus in spontaneous infection: Absence of classical immunologic tolerance. *Proc. Natl. Acad. Sci. USA 69* (1972): 134.

I. Penn and T. E. Starzl. Immunosuppression and cancer. *Transplant. Proc. 5* (1973): 943.

R. T. Prehn. Cancer and the immune response. *Proc. Inst. Med. Chicago 29* (1973): 10.

R. E. Ritts and H. B. Neel. An overview of cancer immunology. *Mayo Clinic Proc. 49* (1974): 118.

F. C. Sparks. Hazards and complications of BCG immunotherapy. *Med. Clin. N.A. 60* (1976): 499.

Symposium on tumor-specific antigens. *Cancer Res. 28* (1968): 1275-1459.

L. Thomas. Reactions to homologous tissue antigens in relation to hypersensitivity. In *Cellular and Humoral Aspects of the Hypersensitive Status* H. S. Lawrence, ed.). Hoeber-Harper, New York, 1959, p. 529.

Epilogue

Cancer: Tomorrow and the Future

No one living today knows and few of us can imagine what the future holds with respect to advances in our knowledge of neoplasia. The possibility of a "magic bullet" such as Salvarsan, the antispirochaetal arsenical of Paul Ehrlich, or penicillin, the antibiotic of Alexander Fleming, seems more remote as our knowledge of the many causes, varied clinical appearances, and unpredictable responses to therapy of cancer increases. Despite the dramatic expansion of our knowledge of fundamental biological processes, medical science has been repeatedly frustrated in its effort to establish a truly effective therapy for the most common forms of malignant neoplasms in the human such as the lung, breast, prostate, and gastrointestinal tract. Yet it is still quite true that our knowledge of the basic nature of the cancer cell can progress no faster than comparable research on the cell and molecular biology of normal cells and tissues. A major question facing us today is: are there the beginnings of knowledge in specific areas of biology that offer promise of significantly expanding our knowledge of the neoplastic transformation and its control in the future? Undoubtedly there are many. The few that are briefly discussed in this epilogue are presented here not for the purpose of prophesying or evangelizing but rather to try to stimulate the reader, be that person young or old, student or professor, layman or professional, to think of the future and what it may hold and to consider seriously the problem of cancer and how it may be solved.

The Future of Cancer Causation:
Cancer Prevention

Within the last 15 years our knowledge of many of the basic mechanisms concerned with the chemical induction of cancer has been increased. Paramount among these discoveries was the demonstration by the Millers and their associates (Chapter 3) that some, if not the vast majority, of chemical carcinogens must first be metabolized to an active form before exerting their carcinogenic effect. Through this discovery the common denominator of almost all the chemical carcinogens was found to be that prior to their action as a carcinogen such chemicals must be converted into a highly reactive molecule capable of modifying the structure of DNA, RNA, protein, and possibly other macromolecules in the cell.

Although this discovery did not elucidate the exact mechanism of the neoplastic transformation, it has been the basis for investigations that may in the future save more human lives by preventing cancer than will ever be saved by the surgeon's knife, the radiotherapists's giant machines, or the medical oncologist's drugs. The topic of which I write is the very real possibility that in the future we may be able to predict the carcinogenic potential of a chemical from a knowledge of its chemical and biochemical reactivity and its metabolic transformations. Already we have seen a significant beginning in this field by the establishment of a rapid assay for the mutagenicity of chemicals or their metabolites employing highly sensitive strains of bacteria, as has been done by Ames and his associates (Chapter 5). Today the Ames test is employed in numerous industrial firms, including pharmaceutical manufacturers, industrial producers of chemicals, and the cosmetics and food industries. New legislation by the federal government has already been enacted requiring that chemical agents to be marketed must first be shown to be reasonably safe in the human environment. While it is clear that the ultimate definition of neoplasia at the present time can be made only in the whole animal, the testing of every new chemical by administration to a large number and varieties of animal species is physically and financially impossible. Rather, as we learn more of the relative carcinogenic potential of specific chemicals, their metabolic reactivity, and their effectiveness as carcinogens in various species in relation to dose, time of administration, and other variables, we will come into a better and better position to predict with reasonable assurance the relative danger as a human carcinogen of specific chemicals that enter our environment.

It is by such means that in the future humans should be better able to control their environment with respect to the number of chemical carcinogens therein, most of which have been placed there by their own ingenuity. Today it is generally accepted that 80% or more of the cases of human cancer can be related to environmental factors. Undoubtedly many of these factors are chemical carcinogens in our environment. Today the future prospects for the prevention of cancer in humans hold a promise as great for future generations as did the development of vaccination and active immunizations for the prevention of infectious disease in the human population almost 200 years ago.

The Natural History and Nature of the Cancer Cell: Future Prospects

Our knowledge of the pathogenesis and natural history of neoplasia has within the last decade increased dramatically not only from the standpoint of basic mechanisms but also, and certainly as important, from the extension of the two-stage hypothesis (Chapter 6) from its original definition in skin to a variety of other organs, including the bone marrow, liver, gastrointestinal tract, and mammary glands. In several of these tissues it is now possible to identify by suitable methodologies the relatively immediate progeny of the initiated cell or cells. In several instances these initiated cell populations can be shown to exist in the organism essentially for an entire lifetime without ever expressing their potential for biological malignancy. Yet the fact that they do possess this potential under the appropriate environmental stimuli has been repeatedly observed. Therefore, if it were possible for us to devise techniques to identify in a reasonable and sufficient manner these populations in the living organism, the potential for scientific gains in our knowledge of the mechanism of tumor promotion as well as the identification of environmental and endogenous promoters for tissues other than the skin would be immense. Furthermore, were it possible to identify such initiated cell populations in many tissues of the human by cytologic, histopathologic, or biochemical means, the early diagnosis and therapy of numerous human cancers could be tremendously simplified. In fact, based on our knowledge of the regression and reversion of specific neoplasms (Chapter 6), appropriate therapy might be devised to eliminate initiated cell populations through their regression or reversion to normal tissue.

The Future Therapy of Cancer

Although this textbook does not consider the therapy of cancer in general, most students of the subject of oncology are vitally interested in and usually have acquired a certain amount of knowledge about the types of therapy utilized for the treatment of human cancer. In general, therapies come under the heading of surgery, radiotherapy, chemotherapy, and most recently, but as yet to a relatively small degree, immunotherapy. While there have clearly been many advances in all of these areas during the past decade, in the author's opinion the most significant advances have been made in the area of chemotherapy. Specifically, multiple drug combinations or so-called combination chemotherapy, used first to treat leukemia and more recently solid tumors, appears at the present time to offer the patient who cannot be further helped by conventional surgery or radiotherapy the greatest chance for years of productive life after the initial diagnosis of the disease. The best examples of success with this type of therapy have been seen in acute lymphatic leukemia in children, where in the best hands 50% of these children will live for 5 years or more and a significant percentage will be totally cured by the use of combination chemotherapy alone. Only 15 years ago the prognosis for this disease was exceedingly bleak, with most patients living less than a year after the diagnosis. A number of other childhood neoplasms such as Wilm's tumor of the kidney, neuroblastoma, and others have a much brighter prognosis as a result of combination drug therapy. Most recently the use of combination chemotherapy in cancer of the breast in women appears to be quite promising.

The major difficulty in the future of combination chemotherapy is that at our present state of knowledge research in this area can be carried out effectively only in the human patient. With the obvious ethical and legal restrictions on human experimentation and the sometimes less obvious administrative restrictions on new drugs, advances in this particular area will necessarily be slow. However, at the present time it is likely that the area of chemotherapy holds the greatest promise for the future of the patient with advanced cancer even on the assumption that no revolutionary new drugs will be forthcoming.

The prevention, nature, and therapy of cancer stand among the major goals of the human race. As long as our world remains relatively peaceful and society struggles for equal prosperity for all humanity, let us hope and pray that future generations will strive to achieve the goals toward which this text is directed.

Index